FOOD
SAFETY

A Reference Handbook

Other Titles in ABC-CLIO's
CONTEMPORARY
WORLD ISSUES
Series

Books in the Contemporary World Issues series address vital issues in today's society such as genetic engineering, pollution, and biodiversity. Written by professional writers, scholars, and nonacademic experts, these books are authoritative, clearly written, up-to-date, and objective. They provide a good starting point for research by high school and college students, scholars, and general readers as well as by legislators, businesspeople, activists, and others.

Each book, carefully organized and easy to use, contains an overview of the subject, a detailed chronology, biographical sketches, facts and data and/or documents and other primary-source material, a directory of organizations and agencies, annotated lists of print and nonprint resources, and an index.

Readers of books in the Contemporary World Issues series will find the information they need in order to have a better understanding of the social, political, environmental, and economic issues facing the world today.

FOOD
SAFETY

A Reference Handbook

Nina E. Redman

**CONTEMPORARY
WORLD ISSUES**

ABC-CLIO

Santa Barbara, California
Denver, Colorado
Oxford, England

Library of Congress Cataloging-in-Publication Data

Redman, Nina.
    Food safety : a reference handbook / Nina E. Redman.
      p.   cm. — (Contemporary world issues)
    Includes bibliographical references and index.
    ISBN 1-57607-158-8 (hardcover : alk paper)
    1. Food adulteration and inspection—Handbooks, manuals, etc. 2. Food industry and trade—Safety measures—Handbooks, manuals, etc. I. Title. II. Series.
TX531.R44   2000
363.19'2—dc21

                                                         00-010427

This book is also available on the World Wide Web as an e-book. Visit www.abc-clio.com for details.

06 05 04 03 02 01 00 10 9 8 7 6 5 4 3 2 1

ABC-CLIO, Inc.
130 Cremona Drive, P.O. Box 1911
Santa Barbara, California 93116-1911

This book is printed on acid-free paper ∞.

Manufactured in the United States of America

*For my grandmother Eleanor Helliwell
and in memory of my grandfather George Helliwell
Thanks for believing in me!*

Contents

Preface

It is estimated that 20 percent of all emergency room visits are due to foodborne illness. As dietary habits change to include more meals prepared away from home, higher consumption of fresh foods, and more imported foods, the risks of foodborne illness change. Food safety procedures that we learned from our parents may not be sufficient to keep us healthy. Food is increasingly contaminated; a steady percentage of chicken, eggs, beef, and pork have some contamination from salmonella and campylobacter. Without taking precautions in the form of safe handling techniques, consumers are almost assured of contracting foodborne illnesses.

Organization

Chapter 1 outlines major issues in food safety today including types of foodborne illnesses, pesticides, antibiotics and growth hormones, irradiation, food disparagement, functional foods, factory farming, regulation, and safe handling guidelines. Chapter 2 is a chronology of important food safety events. Many of these events relate to regulatory changes, foodborne disease outbreaks, and technological changes that impact food safety. Chapter 3 has biographical sketches of prominent people in the food safety field. Improving food safety is a result of the combined efforts of food safety activists, legislators, food technologists, epidemiologists who track the sources of disease, scientists who discover better ways to process food, and companies that dedicate themselves to producing and serving safe food. The people I've chosen are representative of the kinds of people working on food safety today and in the past.

Chapter 4 contains the Food and Drug Administration's Bad Bug Book with current information about foodborne illnesses, causes, statistics, and symptoms. The Center for Science in the Public Interest's guide to food additives is also reproduced, complete with safety recommendations. Chapter 5, Directory of Organizations, includes industry trade groups, activist organizations, and federal, state, and international governmental organizations concerned with food safety. Websites are listed when available. Chapter 6 contains print resources including monographs and periodicals. Materials were chosen based on currency and relevance. Some older materials are included because they're a particularly good source of information. Chapter 7 describes videotapes and databases. Subscription databases for research are presented along with some web-based, free databases. A glossary of frequently used terms is included at the end.

Acknowledgments

I'd like to thank the libraries of the Los Angeles area for their generosity in allowing access to materials, including the Los Angeles Public Library; the Los Angeles County Public Library; the libraries of the University of Southern California including Norris Medical Library; University Research Library at the University of California–Los Angeles; and the library at California Polytechnic University, Pomona.

Thanks to my coworkers at Glendale College Library for their support and encouragement. I especially thank Zohara and Kelly for all those interlibrary loans!

My editor, Alicia Merritt, has been especially helpful and responsive.

My family and friends have offered encouragement and suggestions. My sons, Max and Jackson, have been patient when I've needed to work, and my husband, Steve, has given lots of support and suggestions.

1

Introduction:
A Food Safety Overview

xperts disagree about whether food is safer today than in the past, but they agree that ensuring safe food has become more complex than at any other point in history. Although we have solved many of the food safety challenges of the past, new problems have developed. Before pasteurization of milk, people worried about contracting bovine tuberculosis, brucellosis, and other milk-borne diseases. Today there are concerns about bovine growth hormone, antibiotic, and pesticide residues in milk. Toxic coloring additives used to be added to food unregulated. Now people worry about legal additives and ingredients like Olestra, saccharin, NutraSweet, and hydrogenated oils. Before refrigeration, people used other methods to ensure food safety, including eliminating leftovers by feeding them to their animals. Today proper storage techniques are essential for food safety. A flock of chickens that became diseased one hundred years ago only affected a few people. Now that flocks can be as large as thousands of chickens, an outbreak of salmonella or *campylobacter* can affect many more people. Globalization also affects food safety. The grapes imported during the winter from Chile may have been grown with pesticides that may be illegal in industrialized countries. Setting aside problems of pesticides, the health of the workers picking and processing food directly affects the safety of the product, as do the sanitation practices in the field. Are there toilets and handwashing facilities in the field? Do pickers and processors use them? If not, there is great potential to pass on bacteria, viruses, and parasites.

History

As food safety issues have changed, so has society's methods for making food as safe as possible. Before manufacturing, traditional farming practices and preserving techniques were used to ensure safe food. During the industrial revolution, food began to be processed and packaged. Lacking regulation, manufacturers added whatever they liked to their products. Sweepings from the floor were included in pepper, lead salts were added to candy and cheese, textile inks were used as coloring agents, brick dust was added to cocoa, and copper salts were added to peas and pickles (Borzelleca 1997, 44). In the 1880s women started organizing groups to protest the conditions at slaughterhouses in New York City and adulterated foods, drinks, and drugs in other parts of the country. In 1883, Harvey W. Wiley, chief chemist of the United States Agricultural Department's Bureau of Chemistry, began experimenting with food and drug adulteration. He started a "poison squad," which consisted of human volunteers who took small doses of the poisons used in food preservatives at the time. Wiley worked hard to get legislation passed to regulate what could go into food. Meanwhile, Upton Sinclair spent several weeks in a meatpacking plant investigating labor conditions and turned his discoveries into a book. *The Jungle* by Sinclair was published in 1906. Although the focus of that book was the conditions immigrants experienced in the early twentieth century, there were graphic descriptions of the filth and poor hygiene in packing plants. These descriptions of packing plants—and not the poor working conditions of immigrants—caught the public's attention. People began complaining to Congress and to President Theodore Roosevelt. Pressure was also mounting from foreign governments who wanted some assurances that food imported from the United States was pure and wholesome. Two acts were passed in 1906, the Pure Food and Drug Act and the Beef Inspection Act, to improve food safety conditions.

Regulation only came in response to problems: outbreaks and health hazards were followed by new laws. In 1927 the United States Food, Drug, and Insecticide Administration (now the Food and Drug Administration, or FDA) was created to enforce the Pure Food Act. However, in 1937 over a hundred people died after ingesting a contaminated elixir. The Pure Food and Drug Act proved to have penalties that were too light, and the laws were superseded in 1938 by the Pure Food, Drug, and Cosmetics Act. This act prohibited any food or drug that is dangerous to health to be sold in interstate commerce. The Public Health Service Act of 1944 gave the FDA authority over vaccines and serums and allowed the FDA to inspect restaurants and travel facilities. In 1958 concern over cancer led to the adoption of the Delaney Amendments, which expanded the FDA's regulatory powers to set limits on pesticides and additives. Manufacturers had to prove that additives and pesticides were safe before they could be used. The Fair Packaging and Labeling Act of 1966 standardized the labels of products and required that labels provide honest information. The next major act was the Food Quality Protection Act of 1996. It set new regulations requiring the Hazard Analysis and Critical Control Points (HACCP) system for most food processors. (HACCP, described in detail below, is a process where a manufacturing or processing system is analyzed for potential contamination, and systems are put in place to monitor and control contamination at crucial steps in the manufacturing process.) The act also changed the way acceptable pesticide levels are calculated. Now total exposure from all sources must be calculated.

USDA

Growing in parallel to the FDA was the United States Department of Agriculture (USDA). The USDA is responsible for the safety of most animal products. In the 1890s some European governments raised questions about the safety of U.S. beef. Congress assigned the USDA the task of ensuring that U.S. beef met European standards. In 1891 the USDA started conducting antemortem and postmortem inspections of livestock slaughtered in the United States and intended for U.S. distribution. The USDA began using veterinarians to oversee the inspection process with the goal of preventing diseased animals from entering the food supply.

During World War II more women entered the workforce and consumption of fast food increased. The availability of ready-to-eat foods like processed hams, sausages, soups, hot dogs, frozen dinners, and pizzas increased dramatically. The 1950s saw large growth in meat- and poultry-processing facilities. New ingredients, new technology, and specialization increased the complexity of the slaughter and processing industry. Slaughterhouses went from being small facilities to large plants that used high-speed processing techniques to handle thousands of animals per day. As a result, food technology and microbiology became increasingly important tools to monitor safety. The Food Safety and Inspection Service, the inspection arm of the USDA, grew to more than 7,000 inspectors. But because of the growth in the number of animals slaughtered and processed, it became impossible to individually inspect each carcass. Inspectors must now focus on the production line for compliance, and processing techniques must be strong to compensate for the lack of individual inspection (Schumann 1997, 118).

International Food Safety

Every industrialized country has agencies similar to the FDA and USDA, many with stricter regulations than the United States. In the European Union, food irradiation has been approved for years, genetic engineering is mostly banned, and regulations regarding animal feeds and viral contamination are much more stringent. In less developed countries, the infrastructure needed to impose and enforce regulation is generally lacking, and standards are much more lax. Adulterated food is much more common, and there are many incidents where people have died from tainted products. On an international level, the World Health Organization (WHO), an agency of the United Nations, is very concerned with food safety. In 1983, an expert committee on food safety was convened by the WHO and Food and Agricultural Organization (FAO) of the UN. The committee concluded that illness due to contaminated food is perhaps the most widespread health problem in the contemporary world and an important cause of reduced economic productivity. Foodborne diseases are a major contributor to the estimated 1.5 billion annual episodes of diarrhea in children under five. These diarrheal illnesses cause more than 3 million premature deaths each year. The WHO has many safety-related programs to promote awareness, prevention, and control of food safety risks associated with biological and chemical contamination of foods. It sponsors conferences on topics related to food safety, such as a workshop in 1993 on the health aspects of marker genes in genetically altered plants. It also participates in the Codex Alimentarius Commission established in 1962 jointly with FAO. The purpose of the commission is to establish international standards for food to both ensure food safety and to facilitate trade (World Health Organization 1999). For example, the commission has ruled that beef raised with hormones is safe. Although the European Union does not want to import U.S. beef raised with hormones, it becomes a trade violation if they don't accept it for import.

Food is also regulated at state and local levels. In the United States, individual states regulate agriculture, including the use of pesticides, and state health departments track foodborne diseases. Regulations vary from state to state; some are more stringent than others. County health departments are responsible for inspecting food service establishments and frequently close restaurants that are not complying with health codes.

In addition to public agencies, there are many nongovernmental organizations that are working to improve food safety either through promoting regulation or through research and promotion of improved food safety practices. Safe Tables Our Priority (STOP) was founded as a support and information organization for victims of food poisoning. It was instrumental in getting microbial testing to be part of the 1996 Food Quality Protection Act. Food and Water, a Vermont-based organization, has lobbied extensively for safer food, including working to reduce or ban the use of recombinant bovine growth hormone (rBGH). The American Meat Institute, an organization supported by the beef and poultry industry, does research on food safety and promotes good manufacturing practices and food safety techniques in the industry.

Beyond Regulation

Although manufacturers, processors, and restaurants all want to produce food cheaply and efficiently, they also have strong economic reasons for making safe products. If a product gets recalled as happened with millions of pounds of meat products in 1998 and 1999 following an outbreak of listeriosis, the loss goes far beyond the lost revenue from the unsold product. Consumer confidence in the product must be reestablished before sales will resume their normal level. As Sara J. Lilygren, senior vice-president of the American Meat Institute, an industry trade group, points out, "Brand equity is gold" (Licking 1999).

After the 1993 *E. coli* O157:H7 outbreak in which four children died after eating Jack in the Box hamburgers, the company knew its business would not recover from another serious food safety episode. They implemented a state-of-the-art HACCP system with far more stringent requirements than state and federal regulations. This system included microbial testing that went far beyond what any similar business was doing at the time (Steinauer 1997). Similarly, Odwalla, a juice company, developed much stronger food safety controls after an *E. coli* O157:H7 outbreak was traced to their unpasteurized apple juice. They have worked with farmers and Primus Labs to develop rigorous safety procedures that exceed regulations because their business is based on producing high-quality, safe products. If they sell unwholesome products, the marketplace will put them out of business (McAFee 1998).

Hudson Foods, the company that processed the *E. coli* O157:H7 tainted hamburger that was sold to Jack in the Box restaurants, was dismantled after the incident. But companies do not just react after an outbreak or recall. Food service businesses around the world know that their customers depend on safe food. Nowhere is this more true than in hospitals where dietitians know that many of their food service patrons are immune compromised. Karen Schwartz, director of Food and Nutrition Services at St. Francis Health System in Greenville, South Carolina, notes, "To be sure the food is safe before it gets to us, we tour our primary vendors once a year" (McDermott 1998). A&P supermarkets have made an extensive commitment to HACCP. "We're pursuing HACCP principles on our own simply because it makes good business sense," says Peter Rojek, the corporate director for environmental health for A&P. "We've adopted HACCP principles in monitoring and record keeping. But it's a quality as much as a food safety program, which makes it even more valuable for business" (Lewis 1998).

In Los Angeles, the health department implemented a grading system for restaurants. At inspection, the health inspector goes through a checklist. If 90 to 100 percent of the items are in compliance, the restaurant receives an "A," 80–89 percent is a "B," 70–79 percent is a "C," and anything lower than 70 gets a numeric score. A restaurant that scores less than 60 twice within a year is subject to closure. These grades, on a sign about 8 by 10 inches, must be posted prominently and is usually on a window next to the restaurant's front door.

Restaurants are so anxious to get and keep an A that they have turned to food safety consulting firms for help. National Everclean, based in Calabasas, California, sets up HACCP programs and then conducts surprise inspections to make sure that procedures are being followed. Many of their inspectors are veterans of the health department and know what to look for. Their inspectors deduct points for unsafe conditions and report to restaurant management. Many restaurant managers' bonuses are tied to these scores so there is a lot of incentive to follow safe food practices.

Steritech, based in North Carolina, uses high-tech devices to measure bacterial counts on restaurant surfaces that might otherwise look clean. Steven Grover of the National Restaurant Association says that many restaurants are hiring food safety auditors to protect themselves and their customers. "A lot of companies are now turning to a third party to do what we used to rely on regulatory agencies to do. The government is going to be there after the fact. Our members need someone on their team before an outbreak" (Dickerson 1999). An outbreak is a worst-case scenario, but as people eat more of their meals away from home, they need to be able to depend on the consistent safety of the foods they eat. Restaurants and other food service operations that provide consistently safe food establish consumer confidence and keep or increase their business.

Epidemiology and Foodborne Illnesses

Most of what is known about foodborne illnesses started with epidemiology, the study of disease in a population. John Snow, a London physician, used deductive reasoning, research, and interviews in the 1880s to determine the cause of a cholera epidemic that had killed more than five hundred people in one week. Scientists used Snow's techniques to investigate primarily infectious disease until the 1920s when the field broadened to include clusters of all factors that apply to the incidence of disease among people.

Epidemiological techniques have improved over the years. In the 1970s, Paul Blake developed the case control method. This method compares those who became ill with closely matched individuals who stayed well. By examining what those who became ill did differently from those who stayed well, the source of infection can often be revealed. In the case of foodborne illness, an ill person would be questioned about where and what he ate and matched as closely as possible in age, health status, and eating patterns to someone who stayed well in an effort to pinpoint differences.

In the United States, the Centers for Disease Control and Prevention (CDC) works to help treat and prevent disease at the national level and has increased its scope to lend epidemiological assistance worldwide because of the overlap between the developed and less developed worlds. The people who pick and pack fruits and vegetables in foreign countries that are imported to the United States are handling the U.S. food supply. If foreign workers have illnesses that can be transmitted through food, their illnesses have a direct bearing on our health (Nicols Fox 1997, 30).

Foodborne illness is most often linked to bacteria, but there are actually four agents that can cause foodborne illness: bacteria, viruses, parasites, and prions. Bacterial illness is the most prevalent, but viruses and parasites are being spread through food more commonly than in the past. Prions, small protein strands, have been implicated in Creutzfeldt-Jakob disease. Each type of disease agent has different characteristics that must be considered when implementing food safety strategies.

Bacteria and Food

Bacteria, small microorganisms that do not have a nucleus, can replicate in food, water, or in other environmental media. Some bacteria do not grow well in cold temperatures, while others flourish. Some bacterial strains are extremely virulent, causing infection with as little as two bacteria. Other bacteria must be present in large numbers to cause any problems. The most common way foodborne bacterial illness is transmitted is the fecal-oral route, where fecal matter from an animal or person contaminates foodstuffs. This contamination could result from inadequate hand washing, fecal matter from animals being transferred to meat during the slaughter or processing steps, or even unsterilized manure being used to fertilize crops. Harmful bacteria can also be carried in animals and, even without fecal contamination, can be present in meat or eggs.

One of the most helpful tools scientists have developed to investigate bacterial illnesses is DNA "fingerprinting." Each strain of bacteria has a unique genetic fingerprint. By comparing bacteria from ill persons with bacteria from suspected foods, it is possible to definitively conclude whether that particular food is the causative agent of the disease. This technique has helped health departments tremendously to trace the source of infection and limit outbreaks. The following sections provide specific details about major bacterial illnesses. Please consult Chapter 4 for additional facts and statistics.

Campylobacter

Campylobacter jejuni causes more foodborne illness in the United States than any other bacteria, virus, or parasite, but most people have never heard of it. It was first identified in fetal tissue of aborted sheep in 1913, but it was not isolated from stool samples of patients with diarrhea until 1972. The most common vehicle for transmission today is raw or undercooked poultry, but it can also occur in untreated drinking water, raw milk, and barbecued pork or sausage (Altekruse 1999).

Most cases are relatively minor, causing loose stools. More severe cases result in diarrhea, fever, and abdominal cramping. People who are immune compromised are especially susceptible to getting campylobacteriosis. One study of AIDS patients showed they got the illness at a rate thirty-nine times higher than the general population. Much more rarely (about 1 in 1,000 cases) campylobacter can cause bacteremia (bacteria get into the blood-stream), septic arthritis (bacteria get into the joints and cause stiffening), and Guillaine-Barre syndrome (GBS). GBS starts with fever, malaise, nausea, and muscular weakness. It affects the peripheral nervous system, especially the roots of the spinal cord that face the front of the body. Paralysis follows that may be mild or may require the patient to be placed on a ventilator to avoid respiratory failure. There is no treatment for the disease, besides providing supportive care. Most people recover within a few weeks or months. However, the paralysis can last for many months or even be permanent. Twenty percent of victims have a permanent disability and 5 percent die of GBS (Altekruse 1999).

Reiter's syndrome, a form of infectious arthritis, is some-times caused by campylobacter. Generally affecting older people, it causes pain and swelling of the joints and tendons and inflammation of the tendons. Typically, it occurs in discrete episodes that last weeks to months. It may disappear after one episode or it may recur and become a chronic illness.

Although the number of cases of campylobacteriosis that result in serious illnesses like Reiter's syndrome and GBS are less than 1 percent of all cases, the large number of people that contract the illness each year (over 2 million in the United States alone) means that thousands (20,000 each year in the United States) will suffer serious results (Altekruse 1999).

A 1995 study by the USDA showed 98 percent of poultry tested was contaminated with campylobacter. Campylobacter lives in the intestines of chickens without causing any harm to the chicken. Meat becomes contaminated when it comes in contact with fecal matter from chickens. Because chickens live in close quarters today with flocks as large as tens of thousands of birds, an infection of campylobacteriosis can easily spread to other chickens. Most of the disease is spread, however, during the transportation and slaughter steps. With assembly-line processing, the carcasses are handled together, which results in cross-contamination. In one study, bacteria counts increased up to 1,000 percent from the time the chickens left the farm to the time they were packaged (Nicols Fox 1997, 195).

Recent legislation improving food safety in chicken processing plants may be starting to show some results. A 15 percent decline in the number of campylobacter-related illnesses was reported between 1997 and 1998 according to the CDC. Both the USDA and the FDA have instituted regulations requiring HACCP programs (DeNoon 1999). However, consumers must continue to be vigilant to prevent illness.

Listeria

Listeria monocytogenes was discovered in the 1920s. It is a particularly pernicious bacteria found in soil and water that can survive refrigerator temperatures and even freezing. It can be found on some vegetables as well as on meat and dairy products. In 1998 an outbreak was traced to hot dogs and other processed meats from the Bill Mar plant in Zeeland, Michigan. Sara Lee, the parent company, voluntarily recalled 30 million pounds of meat.

Because heat kills listeria, it is most often associated with ready-to-eat foods. In the United States, 1,850 cases of listeriosis, the disease *Listeria monocytogenes* causes, are reported annually.

Many more people probably get the disease but in a form so mild they are never diagnosed and treated. The bacteria can live easily in the intestinal tract of animals without harming them, and it has been found in at least thirty-seven mammalian species, both domestic and feral. Some studies suggest that 1 to 10 percent of humans may be intestinal carriers of *Listeria monocytogenes* (United States Food and Drug Administration 1999).

Listeria can cause septicemia, meningitis, encephalitis, and intrauterine or cervical infections in pregnant women that may cause miscarriages or stillbirths. It appears to be able to pass through the placenta to the child, so that even if an infected child survives childbirth, it may die shortly after birth. The symptoms of listeriosis are usually influenza-like, including chills and fever. Listeriosis may also cause gastrointestinal symptoms such as nausea, vomiting, and diarrhea. One of the challenges of tracing sources of the bacteria is the relatively long incubation period. Many cases take weeks to show up, increasing the range of possible tainted foods.

Of the 1,850 cases reported annually in the United States, about 425 are fatal. If the disease is caught early enough, it can be easily treated with antibiotics. The people most at risk are AIDS patients who contract listeriosis at three hundred times the rate of people with normal immune systems. People with cancer or kidney disease and the elderly also have increased risk. Pregnant women are twenty times more likely to get the disease, but it is their infants in utero that suffer the serious effects of the disease. Healthy adults and children occasionally get infected with listeria, but it rarely turns into serious illness (United States Food and Drug Administration 1999).

The last two major outbreaks in the United States came from processed meats, when 17 died in 1998 (Spake 1999), and soft Mexican cheese in the 1980s, when 142 contracted the disease and 46 died (Nicols Fox 1997, 274). Vegetables grown in soil contaminated with listeria (probably from manure in fertilizer) are another common carrier of the bacteria. Ready-to-eat foods are often consumed without further cooking. Although processed food is generally pasteurized, if there are problems at the processing plant, the food can become contaminated after pasteurization.

Foods that are not pasteurized can be a source of contamination also. Two people died in France in 1998 from eating cheese made from raw milk. Many northern European countries require that cheeses only be made from pasteurized milk, but over half of France's 350 kinds of cheese are made with raw milk. The French government has heightened inspection by increased sampling of raw milk cheeses. If any bacteria are found, the cheese is discarded. Due to the stricter regulations and frequent inspections, France has cut the number of cases by two-thirds, down to 225 who got sick because of listeria in 1997 (Sicakyuz 1999).

To avoid illness from listeria, immune compromised people should avoid packaged meats unless they are served steaming hot and avoid soft cheeses like Brie, Camembert, blue-veined cheeses, and Mexican-style cheese. As of 1999, the USDA's Hazard Analysis and Critical Control Points regulations do not require microbial testing for processed foods. Bills before Congress would change that and strengthen the USDA's ability to order a recall of affected products (Licking and Carey 1999).

Salmonella

Salmonella is the second most common source of food poisoning in the United States after campylobacter. It generally causes sudden headache, diarrhea, nausea, and vomiting, and the illness often persists for several days. Symptoms may be minor or severe, causing dehydration or even death. The CDC estimates salmonella causes 1,000 to 2,000 deaths in the United States each year (United States Food and Drug Administration 1999).

Salmonella is most often associated with raw eggs and undercooked poultry. A 1990 USDA study found 57 percent of chickens were contaminated with the bacteria (Puzo 1990). Better handling techniques that were implemented in 1997 reduced that number to 16 percent in 1998 ("Reflects HACCP 'Payoff'" 1999). The bacteria live harmlessly in the intestines of chickens. During the slaughter and processing steps, the bacteria often contaminate the carcasses. Eggshells are wiped with an antibacterial agent to rid them of salmonella contamination, but ironically this also removes the protective coating on the egg, which allows the salmonella bacteria to penetrate the shell (Waltner-Toews 1992, 53).

In 1999 alfalfa sprouts were implicated in an outbreak of salmonellosis centered in Oregon and Washington where twenty-one people became ill. The seeds had become contaminated with the bacteria. Salmonella has also contaminated other fruits and vegetables, including tomatoes, cantaloupes, and fresh orange juice, although most cases are caused by raw or undercooked eggs. A major outbreak was isolated to ice cream in 1994, when the CDC estimated 224,000 developed salmonellosis. Although the company used no eggs in its products, independent contractors who delivered the milk to the plant backhauled eggs in the trucks without properly washing the trucks between loads. The company had to recall the ice cream and subsequently purchased its own trucks to ensure product safety (Nicols Fox 1997, 175–177).

Interestingly, salmonellosis is very uncommon in the developing world where diarrheal illnesses are very common. The people eat almost exclusively locally grown food, which makes salmonella much less likely to spread and contaminate other foods. By contrast, the rate of salmonella poisoning was sharply up from 1950 until the late 1990s in the Western world (Nicols Fox 1997, 182).

There are signs that salmonella poisoning may have started to decline, however. Cases were down 44 percent for *Salmonella enteritidis*, the type of salmonella associated with eggs (DeNoon 1999), and there is hope for a vaccine in the future. Scientists at the University of California–Santa Barbara have discovered that salmonella bacteria carry a gene, called "dam," that serves as an on/off switch for a variety of weapons used by the bacteria to produce disease when it infects humans. If the bacteria do not have the dam gene, it will provoke an immune response, and therefore could be used as a vaccine. Mice were immunized with the dam-less salmonella and all survived a dose of pathogenic *Salmonella typhimurium*, 50,000 times the normal dose required to kill at least half the animals.

The dam gene is also found in many other harmful bacteria, including *Vibrio cholerae* (which causes cholera), *Yersinia pestis* (which causes plague), shigella, *Haemophilus influenzae* (which causes meningitis), and the bacteria that cause syphilis. It will take a long time to produce a vaccine that is safe for humans, but the vaccine could be used to treat cattle and chickens. If those animals were no longer able to host the bacteria, it would significantly improve the safety of the food supply (Maugh 1999).

E. coli O157:H7

Escherichia coli is a type of bacteria that thrives in our intestines and helps digest food. Most strains are beneficial, but a few release harmful toxins that can cause great discomfort and even death. *E. coli* O157:H7 was first isolated in 1982 when forty-seven people in Michigan and Oregon became violently ill (Koutkia 1997). The bacterium contained a few strands of genetic material that caused it to produce a shigella-type toxin. Scientists believe the toxin first destroys blood vessels in the intestines, causing bloody diarrhea. Bloody diarrhea is the most telling symptom of this type of *E. coli* infection. Most people experience bloody diarrhea and abdominal pain and recover, but about 6 percent develop hemolytic uremic syndrome (HUS). Although rare up until the 1980s, HUS is a disease of the blood and kidneys that is now the leading cause of kidney failure in U.S. and Canadian children (Nicols Fox 1997, 213). HUS develops when the toxin penetrates the intestinal wall and passes into the bloodstream. Once in the bloodstream, the toxin damages vessels throughout the body.

When the *E. coli* toxins enter the bloodstream, they shred cells. The debris clogs the kidneys. After the kidneys fail, other organs are affected, including the heart, lungs, and central nervous system. There is no cure. In fact, treatment with antibiotics is thought to exacerbate the condition because the antibiotics kill other beneficial bacteria, leaving more resources for the *E. coli* O157:H7. It can also weaken the toxic *E. coli* bacteria, causing the release of more toxins. Only the symptoms of the disease can be treated; the kidneys can be supported with dialysis and damaged organs can be repaired. About 5 percent of people who contract HUS die, and many survivors of the disease are left with diabetes, kidney damage, visual impairment, or a colostomy (Kluger 1998).

E. coli O157:H7 is most commonly associated with cattle. It does not harm the 1 to 2 percent of cattle that carry the bacteria in their gut (Koutkia 1997). Transmission of the bacteria can occur during the slaughter process. Sometimes fecal matter from the intestines contaminates the meat. If the meat is ground to make hamburger, the bacteria spread throughout the meat. Since most meat made into hamburger is pooled from many animals, contamination from one carcass can infect large batches of meat. Heat kills the bacteria. If a steak is contaminated, it will only be contaminated on the edges. The bacteria will be destroyed in the cooking process, even if the steak is not cooked all the way through. Since contamination can occur throughout the entire hamburger patty, a burger must be thoroughly cooked and reach an internal temperature of 160 degrees F to be safe.

The bacteria can also be transmitted in other ways. Water contaminated with cattle feces has been implicated in several outbreaks of infection caused by *E. coli* O157:H7 that were traced to fruits and vegetables. Unpasteurized milk can also be a source of the strain. Occasionally cattle feces get into a municipal water supply. At daycare centers, usually one child gets the infection and spreads it to the other children. Altogether the CDC estimates that 20,000 people in the United States become ill from *E. coli* O157:H7, and of those, 250 die, mostly children and the elderly (Kluger 1998).

Perhaps the most highly publicized outbreak of *E. coli* contamination occurred in hamburgers served at Jack in the Box restaurants. Five hundred people became ill and four children died. The largest outbreak occurred in Japan in 1996 when radishes were contaminated. Over 9,500 people became ill and twelve children died. Most *E. coli* O157:H7 contamination occurs during the summer months—perhaps because people are more likely to eat at backyard barbecues and eat more fruits and vegetables.

Fortunately, scientists are discovering ways to eliminate or at least reduce *E. coli* O157:H7 contamination. A joint research team of the USDA and Cornell University has discovered that cattle fed a grain diet, such as corn, instead of hay or grass, harbor three hundred times *more E. coli* O157:H7 bacteria in their intestines. The bacteria from the grain-fed cows were also much more likely to survive a one-hour bath in an acid similar to that in a human stomach. While 80 percent of the bacteria from the grain-fed cows survived the acid bath, virtually all the bacteria from the hay-fed group were killed in the acid bath. It appears that the digestive tracts of cattle have a difficult time breaking down starch. Therefore, large amounts of grain can pass into the cows' intestines undigested. This in turn triggers fermentation that provides nutrients for the *E. coli* to grow on, and the environment also favors acid-resistant strains. Scientists speculate that switching the diet of cows in the last few weeks before slaughter could greatly reduce the *E. coli* O157:H7 levels in the intestines and therefore reduce harmful effects from fecal contamination if it occurs (Couzin 1998).

Other researchers at the National Institutes of Health have been working to develop a vaccine against *E. coli* O157:H7 that could be administered to cattle or to people. Clinical trials have been conducted on adults, and trials are being considered for young children. It's not clear whether the vaccine will work in cattle because antibodies may not be able to reach the bacteria. In cattle, the *E. coli* O157:H7 bacteria swim freely in the intestine instead of attaching to the intestinal wall as they do in humans. Since antibodies circulate in the bloodstream, the intestinal wall receives the antibodies, but the contents of the intestine do not. Another approach being studied involves feeding cattle harmless strains of *E. coli* that are believed to inhibit growth of the O157:H7 strain. In addition, tighter controls on beef slaughtering and processing facilities, including more microbial testing, steam vacuum treatment of carcasses, and irradiation, can all reduce contamination levels (Couzin 1998).

Shigella

Shigella causes a little less than 10 percent of all foodborne illness in the United States. It is widespread worldwide and is very virulent: as little as ten cells can cause infection. Shigellosis (the disease caused by shigella) usually strikes between twelve and fifty hours after the contaminated food is consumed. It can cause abdominal pain, cramps, diarrhea, fever, and vomiting. On rare occasions it can cause Reiter's disease, reactive arthritis, and hemolytic uremic syndrome. It is often found in prepared salads, raw vegetables, milk, other dairy products, and poultry (United States Food and Drug Administration 1999).

Yersinia

There are three pathogenic species of yersinia. *Y. pestis* causes the plague and is not transmitted through food. *Y. entercolitica* and *Y. pseudotuberculosis* cause gastrointestinal problems including abdominal pain, diarrhea, and vomiting. Yersinia infections often mimic appendicitis and can sometimes result in unnecessary surgery. The bacteria can also cause infections in wounds, joints, and the urinary tract. *Y. pseudotuberculosis* is very rare in the United States but occurs more frequently in Japan, Scandinavia, and other parts of northern Europe. Strains of *Y. entercolitica* can be found in meats, including beef, pork, lamb, oysters and fish, and also in raw milk. Although most people recover quickly from yersiniosis, about 2 to 3 percent develop reactive arthritis (United States Food and Drug Administration 1999).

Staphylococcus

Foods that require lots of handling during preparation and are kept at slightly elevated temperatures after preparation, including prepared salads like egg, tuna, macaroni, potato, and chicken salad and bakery products like cream-filled pastries, are frequently carriers of staphylococcus. It can also appear in meats, poultry, and dairy products. Staphylococcus are present in the nasal passages and throats and on the hair and skin of 50 percent or more of all healthy individuals. The rate is even higher among hospital workers. Staphylococcus can also survive in air, dust, sewage, water, milk, food equipment, and environmental surfaces. Because it is so prevalent, it is difficult to prevent transmission even with careful handling practices. The most usual course of Staphylococcal food poisoning is very rapid onset of symptoms, including nausea, vomiting, and abdominal cramping. This generally lasts about two days. Although the number of reported cases is relatively low (usually less than 10,000 per year in the United States), the actual number is probably much higher since many cases go unreported because the duration of the illness is very short, and the symptoms are not that severe (United States Food and Drug Administration 1999).

Parasites

Parasites, small microscopic animals that need a host to survive, are transmitted through the fecal-oral route. They live in the intestines of humans and other animal hosts. They are excreted in the feces and they spread through feces-contaminated water, contaminated water on produce, manure used as fertilizer, carcasses that become contaminated during the slaughter process, and poor personal hygiene of food handlers. Unlike bacteria, which often take large numbers to cause infection, a single parasite can cause illness. Since parasites are relatively stable in the environment, difficult to kill, and food processing and storage techniques that discourage bacteria have little effect, they are challenging to eliminate from food (Jaykus 1997).

Perhaps the best known parasite in the United States is *Trichinella spiralis*, a small roundworm found in raw pork that causes trichinosis. The life cycle of *T. spiralis* is similar to many other parasitic infections: a human eats undercooked pork and also unknowingly ingests the encapsulated larvae of the parasite.

The coating is digested in the stomach and small intestine, freeing the larvae to invade the lining of the small intestine. They become adults within a week. Sometimes the adult worm deposits larvae in the lymphatic system where the larvae enter the bloodstream and can thus be spread throughout the body. Usually the larvae concentrate in the muscles of the diaphragm, eyes, neck, throat, larynx, and tongue. Eventually, the larvae capsules become calcified. Very few infected people have sufficient symptoms to recognize the disease. Early symptoms include diarrhea, vomiting, and nausea. These can be followed by pain, stiffness, swelling of muscles, and swelling in the face. Thiabendazole effectively kills the parasites in the digestive tract, and anti-inflammatory drugs can ease the symptoms (United States Food and Drug Administration 1999).

Although trichinella has been well understood for years, it does not cause as much foodborne illness as three other parasites: *Giardia lamblia*, *Cryptosporidium parvum*, and *Cyclospora*. These waterborne parasites can be transferred to food from infected food handlers or if contaminated water is used to irrigate or wash fruits or vegetables. Five outbreaks of giardiasis have been traced to food contamination from infected food handlers. The organism prefers moist, cool conditions. The largest foodborne outbreak of giardiasis occurred when twenty-four out of thirty-six people who consumed macaroni salad at a picnic became ill. The disease causes diarrhea that generally lasts one to two weeks. However, it can become chronic and last for months or even years. If it does become chronic, it is difficult to treat (United States Food and Drug Administration 1999).

Cryptosporidium infects many herd animals, such as cows, goats, and sheep, and has also caused outbreaks in apple cider and homemade chicken salad. It usually causes watery diarrhea that lasts two to four days, but it can also cause coughing and low-grade fever accompanied by severe intestinal distress. After conducting studies using blood analysis techniques, experts concluded that 80 percent of the population in North America has had cryptosporidiosis. Although it is a relatively minor problem for most healthy individuals, it can be fatal to immune compromised populations such as AIDS patients (United States Food and Drug Administration 1999).

Cyclospora cayentanensis is a one-celled parasite that was first discovered in 1977. It caused a major outbreak in 1996 affecting over 1,400 people that was traced to raspberries imported from Guatemala and fresh basil. The berries were most likely contaminated when they were sprayed with insecticides or fungicide that was mixed with water containing the parasites' eggs, called oocysts. The parasite causes watery diarrhea and intestinal cramps that can last for weeks. It generally takes about one week from infection for symptoms to appear and can be treated with sulfa drugs. Typically symptoms go away and then return. The parasite tends to appear most frequently on produce. Washing produce can help, but usually does not completely eliminate the problem. Some delicate fruits, such as raspberries, have many crevices that the oocysts can stick to (United States Food and Drug Administration 1999).

Another source of parasites is raw seafood. The Japanese suffer from high rates of nematode infection resulting from high rates of consumption of raw fish. It occurs less frequently in the United States where raw fish consumption is moderate. One of the worms, *Eustronglyides* sp., can be seen with the naked eye and causes septicemia. Other worms are much smaller. Well-trained sushi chefs are good at spotting the large parasites, but other techniques are necessary to protect against the smaller ones.

Blast freezing is one of the techniques that kills parasites. The USDA Retail Food Code requires freezing for all fish that will be consumed raw. The exception is tuna, which rarely contains parasites. Often fish get parasites from eating smaller fish that have the parasites. Fish raised in captivity and fed fish pellets rarely have parasites. High acid marinades do not affect parasites, so they should not be used as a substitute for cooking or freezing (Parseghian 1997).

Viruses

Viruses, like parasites, pose great problems for food safety because they are environmentally stable, they are resistant to many of the traditional methods used to control bacteria, and a very small amount of a virus can cause infection. This means that virtually any food can serve as a vehicle for transmission. Viral gastroenteritis was reported as the most common foodborne illness in Minnesota from 1984 to 1991. It's not clear just how pervasive foodborne viral illnesses are, partly because viruses are difficult to test for (Jaykus 1997).

Hepatitis A

The most common viral diseases spread by food are hepatitis A and Norwalk virus. Hepatitis A is a relatively mild hepatitis that causes a sudden onset of fever, malaise, nausea, abdominal discomfort, and loss of appetite, followed by several days of jaundice. Hepatitis A virus is excreted in the feces of infected people, and contamination can occur if food handlers are not rigorous about personal hygiene. Cold cuts and sandwiches, fruit and fruit juices, milk and dairy products, as well as vegetables, salads, shellfish, and iced drinks, have often been implicated in outbreaks. The incubation period of ten to fifty days is so long that it can be difficult to locate the source of infection. It is also communicable between individuals, making it hard to know whether the transmission was person-to-person contact or foodborne. The incidence of disease in developing countries is not particularly high because most people are exposed to the disease in childhood and develop immunity (United States Food and Drug Administration 1999).

Norwalk Virus

Norwalk virus is a mild, self-limiting gastroenteritis causing nausea, vomiting, diarrhea, and abdominal pain. It is generally associated with shellfish and salad ingredients. Raw or inadequately steamed oysters and clams are often associated with Norwalk virus. Experts estimate that one-third of viral gastroenteritis is caused by Norwalk virus. Symptoms generally develop 24–48 hours after consuming contaminated food and last 24–60 hours. Complications are rare (United States Food and Drug Administration 1999).

Mad Cow Disease

Bovine spongiform encephalopathy (BSE) is a disease that strikes cows, causing them to develop spongy areas in their brains and suffer personality disorders. When the disease was first noticed in Britain in 1986, some cows were found staggering around in circles, hence the name, *mad cow disease*. As of 1999, more than 173,000 cows had been diagnosed with the disease and more than 4 million had been destroyed in an attempt to wipe out the disease (Blakeslee 1999). In addition to the toll on cattle, humans began developing a related disease, Creutzfeldt-Jakob disease, at earlier ages than normal and in increasing numbers and severity.

Creutzfeldt-Jakob disease (CJD) was first described in the 1920s by Hans Gerhard Creutzfeldt and Alfons Jakob. Symptoms can include loss of coordination, personality changes, mania, and dementia. People usually die within a year or two of diagnosis. It generally affects about one in 1 million people age 50 or older through spontaneous means or as an inherited condition. Very rarely, it has been contracted through infected tissues that were transplanted, such as corneas, from contaminated surgical instruments, or by injection of growth hormones that were derived from CJD-infected pituitary extracts. In 1995 scientists in Britain identified a new type of CJD called new variant CJD (nvCJD). This new type struck mostly younger people and the brain tissue of these victims looks exactly like the brain tissue of cows that die of BSE.

As epidemiologists studied nvCJD, they began to suspect a species-to-species transfer was taking place. People who had consumed brain or spinal tissue from cows were getting the disease. The incubation period of the disease may be as long as twenty to twenty-five years according to Simon Cousens, an epidemiologist at the London School of Hygiene and Tropical Medicine. As of early 1999, thirty-nine people had died from nvCJD, and it is unclear whether the epidemic is almost over or on an upswing. With the long incubation period, scientists aren't sure how many people will be affected. Estimates range from a few hundred to as many as 80,000 ("Cull Maff" 1998). It seems likely that the cows got the disease from eating sheep brains contaminated with scrapie, a similar disease found in sheep. Sheep's brain tissue is rendered into cattle feed.

No one is sure exactly how BSE is transmitted to humans. Some scientists believe it is a virus that has yet to be discovered, while others believe it is caused by a deformed protein molecule, called a prion, that attaches to a healthy protein molecule and deforms it. The two molecules then split apart and go on to attack other healthy protein molecules. The prion is resistant to common sterilization methods including bleach, boiling, alcohol, exposure to chemical agents, and irradiation. Even after burning infected tissue, the prion could still be detected in the ashes. In a test on cows, as little as one-quarter of a teaspoon of the transmission agent given as feed caused BSE (Waverly 1998).

The primary reason this disease spread was the inclusion of rendered animal protein in feed. In order to raise cattle quickly, it is necessary to feed them large amounts of protein. Proteins derived from vegetables are less dense and can be more expensive than rendered animal proteins. Cows fed grass, hay, alfalfa, and other forage produce just ten to fifty pounds of milk per day, whereas cows given supplements of animal fats, bone meal, blood, and meat protein can produce as much as 130 pounds per day. From 1987 to 1996 the number of dairy cows in the U.S. dropped by 11 percent while production increased 8 percent due to breeding, hormones, drugs, and specialized feeds. In Britain, where there is less farming of hay and other grains for cattle, it is estimated that cows received as much as four pounds per day of rendered animal protein. These animal products are derived from sick, diseased animals and leftovers from the slaughterhouses. For example, the backbones and heads of cattle are sent to the rendering plant where they are boiled and ground up and then sold as animal protein. This amounts to cannibalism for the cows. Human cannibalism can lead to transmissible spongiform encephalopathy (TSE), similar to CJD, called kuru.

Exacerbating the cannibalism is the use of low-temperature vacuum systems in the rendering process. Since water boils at any temperature when in a vacuum, some rendering plants switched to this system to save energy costs because they could use room-temperature water instead of heating it. It is estimated that 60 to 70 percent of British plants switched to this system in the 1980s. In the United States one-quarter to one-third of plants use the low-temperature process. Although boiling (212 degrees F, or 100 degrees C at sea level) does not eradicate BSE completely, the amount of infectious agent is reduced considerably using the regular processing method but not at all with the low-temperature vacuum process (Shell 1998).

Although no one in the United States has been diagnosed with nvCJD yet, there is concern that it could happen. Cows in the United States sometimes become "downer cows," going lame and becoming unable to stand. These cows become sick for a variety of reasons, including broken legs and "milk fever," but some may have a form of BSE. In 1985 an outbreak of encephalopathy in minks raised for clothing occurred in Stetsonville, Wisconsin. Richard Nash, a scientist at the University of Wisconsin School of Veterinary Medicine, investigated the outbreak and found that the mink had been fed slaughtered animals including about 95 percent downer dairy cows. Marsh tested his hypothesis that the downer cows had transmitted the infection by injecting two six-week-old calves with mink brain from the farm. The calves developed the neurological disease eighteen and nineteen months after inoculation and had spongiform degeneration at necropsy. The disease was also transmissible back to mink by injection or by feeding the brain tissue to the animals (Fox 1997, 311). This led Marsh to conclude that the United States may have its own form of BSE, perhaps disguised in downer cows. Although downer cows may not be added directly to the food supply without clearance from a veterinarian, occasionally some do get into the human meat supply; the remainder are fed back to cattle and other animals through the rendering process.

About 1 million cattle brains are consumed annually in the United States. In addition to the cattle brains people eat intentionally, some brain tissue often gets into other meat products. Pneumatic stun guns were used until recently to stun cows before slaughter. The stun gun spread brain tissue to other organs. When mechanical deboning is done, the spinal column is squeezed and plucked to get the last bits of meat off. In this way spinal column tissue can get into hamburger and bologna. In May 1997, inspectors for the Food Safety Inspection Service were told to report facilities where brain and spinal cord might be getting into meat. Although no nvCJD has been diagnosed in North America, it's possible that other types of TSE with different symptoms are appearing in the United States and are diagnosed as spontaneously occurring forms of dementia (Shell 1998).

Other Food Safety Threats

Besides bacteria, viruses, and parasites, there are other potential sources of foodborne illness, including pesticides, hormones in milk and cattle, overuse of antibiotics in farm animals, genetically engineered plants, food additives, and naturally occurring contaminants. In order to evaluate the safety of these sometimes controversial farming and manufacturing methods, scientists and policymakers use a tool called risk assessment.

Risk assessment is a formal extension of the type of analysis each of us does every day when we take risks such as driving a car, walking across the street, using an old stove, exercising, or playing sports. Even though these things pose small risks of injury or death, we take those risks because the benefits of the activities—getting to where we want to go, eating hot food, enjoying ourselves—are high compared to the relatively small chance of harm. Foods pose similar risks. There are several types of food risks. Eating too much of certain types of foods, such as fats, can be harmful. Eating spoiled or contaminated food can be very dangerous, even deadly. Pesticides and food additives can also pose risks. Risk assessment is the process of evaluating the risks posed and determining whether a food ingredient or pesticide can safely be consumed in the amounts likely to be present in a given food.

In order to compute risks, scientists must consider both the probability and the impact of contracting the disease. A disease with high probability, but little impact, is of less concern than a disease with high probability and high impact. The object is to either reduce the probability of contracting the disease or the severity of impact. Either action will reduce risk. To evaluate risks, a four-step process is used: hazard identification, exposure assessment, dose-response assessment, and risk characterization.

During the first step, hazard identification, an association between a disease and the presence of a pathogen in a food is documented. For example, contracting dysentery is associated with eating chickens contaminated with campylobacter. Information may be collected about conditions under which the pathogen survives, grows, causes infection, and dies. Data from epidemiological studies are used along with surveillance data, challenge testing, and studies of the pathogen.

After the hazard is identified, exposure is assessed. This step examines the ways in which the pathogen is introduced, distributed, and challenged during production, distribution, and consumption of food. Exposure assessment takes the hazard from general identification to a specific process-related exposure. For example, chickens might become exposed to campylobacter by drinking unchlorinated water or from contact with other chickens on the farm, the carcass might be exposed during defeathering or on the processing line, the amount of campylobacter may be reduced in number during the chilling step and increased in number during the packaging step. In this way, the pathogen population can be traced and the likelihood of it reaching the consumer can be estimated.

The third step, dose-response assessment, determines what health result is likely to occur when the consumer is exposed to the pathogen population determined in the exposure assessment step. This step can be very difficult because there are often not good data about what levels of pathogen exposure have health consequences. Another significant factor is the strength of the immune system of the particular consumer. Immune compromised populations such as young children, the elderly, AIDS patients, and chemotherapy patients may react to lower exposure levels and have more severe health consequences.

Risk characterization, the final step, integrates the information from the previous steps to determine the risk to various populations and particular types of consumers, for example, children in general and children who consume three or more glasses of apple juice per day. Computer modeling techniques are often used in this step to ease the computational burden of trying many different scenarios (Lammerding and Paoli 1997). With so many variables, risk assessment does not produce exact, unequivocal results. At best it produces good estimates of the impact of a given pathogen on a population, at worst it over- or underestimates the impact.

Pesticides

The U.S. Federal Insecticide, Fungicide, and Rodenticide Act (FIFRA) defines pesticides as "any substance or mixture of substances intended for preventing, repelling, or mitigating any insects, rodents, nematodes, or fungi, or any other forms of life declared to be pests." This also includes substances or mixtures intended for use as plant regulators, defoliants, or desiccants. Pesticides are an integral part of agricultural practice in the United States, and 35 to 45 percent of all pesticides produced worldwide are used in the United States.

With over 1,400 active chemical ingredients and over 60,000 chemical formulations, it is impossible to know with certainty what the long-term effects, if any, will be on human health. Pesticides can be naturally occurring substances such as nicotine, pyrethrum (found in chrysanthemums), hellebore, rotenone, and camphor, or synthetically produced inorganic chemicals, metals, metallic salts, organophosphates, carbamates, and halogenated hydrocarbons (Borzelleca 1997).

Pesticides work in many different ways to kill pests. Stomach poisons attack chewing insects such as ants, flies, grasshoppers, and crickets. In-contact poisons kill pests when they touch the poison, fumigants kill when the substance is breathed by the pest, and residual poisons attack when they are applied to the surface of pests. Some pesticides inhibit metabolic function or reproduction of pests, some mimic hormones, some destroy cells, and some are physical poisons that kill cells indiscriminantly by physical means such as suffocation. Unfortunately, most pesticides are not selective and affect the same target organ in the pest, the plant the farmer is raising, and nontarget species such as people and animals (Borzelleca 1997). Pesticides also tend to concentrate. In an experiment on dichlorodiphenyl-trichloroethane (DDT), DDT was applied to a lake at .02 parts per million (PPM). Within a year plankton showed DDT concentrations of 10 PPM, little fish showed 900 PPM, and fish-eating birds showed 2,000 PPM. Pesticides accumulate in fatty tissue in animals, and the runoff from pesticides gets into groundwater (Waltner-Toews 1992).

Before a company can market a pesticide in the United States, it must demonstrate to the Food and Drug Administration that it is safe. The FDA determines what concentration levels of a pesticide or its breakdown products are safe. The tolerance levels, the amount allowed to be present on food at harvest, were adjusted by the 1996 Food Quality Protection Act to be based on what levels are safe for children. The FDA sets these levels by studying toxicological data and safety field trials, and by considering the economic impact of the use of the pesticide. Some of the questions it considers are: What happens to the chemical during processing? Does the chemical concentration break down? Are the new products it forms safe? The FDA also uses total diet studies, where foods are gathered from a complete daily diet, chemically analyzed, and the total diet is compared to tolerance levels for various chemicals. These studies can be quite helpful because pesticide levels are often reduced during processing, refining, storage, and food preparation. Therefore the total effect of pesticides might aggregate to unsafe levels, or might be significantly mitigated by the other processing steps.

Although the FDA and Environmental Protection Agency (EPA) regulate pesticides used in this country, one of the most disturbing aspects of pesticide production is that pesticides that have been banned from *use* in the United States continue to be *manufactured* in the United States and sold abroad. In many less developed countries, the regulatory infrastructure doesn't exist to require testing, labeling, and product review of imported pesticides. Pesticide poisoning is common among farmworkers, and ironically many of the pesticides come back to the United States in the form of residues on imported produce.

No valid human epidemiological studies have established a positive correlation between consumption of pesticide residues in food and adverse health effects. However, farmworkers experience higher rates of cancer than other groups, indicating that at high levels of exposure, there are significant risks. A prudent pesticide strategy must include an evaluation of need and consider the following:

1. The smallest amount of the pesticide to use (or none at all)
2. The safety of production workers and applicators of the pesticide
3. The safety of consumers of the product, including potentially sensitive segments of the population
4. The interactions of pesticides with other chemicals, including drugs, nutrients, and other chemicals
5. Environmental and ecological concerns, including groundwater and surface water contamination and effects on wildlife
6. Persistence—how long it stays in the environment
7. Bioaccumulation—how it concentrates in species other than the target, as illustrated above by the DDT experiment, and how it might alter the balance of nature.

There are also risk-benefit considerations, including the economic aspects of increasing food production per acre, decreasing food losses during storage, and destroying vectors of disease, such as the aflatoxins that grow on untreated peanuts. Pesticides require careful, judicious study so that they can be used safely (Borzelleca 1997).

Alar, Oprah, and Food Disparagement Laws

In 1989, *60 Minutes* broadcast a report, "A Is for Apple," about the use of Alar, a growth regulator used on apples. The Environmental Defense Fund had prepared a report showing that Alar was extremely dangerous and would result in increased numbers of cancer deaths in children. Apple sales fell and many school lunch programs stopped offering apples that had been treated with Alar.

The EPA started proceedings to ban Alar, but the manufacturer, Uniroyal, decided to pull Alar from the market. A number of apple growers sued the Environmental Defense Fund and CBS, the producer of *60 Minutes*. The case against the Environmental Defense Fund was dismissed and the apple growers lost their case against CBS. After the lawsuit, thirteen states enacted food disparagement laws. These laws essentially extend libel laws, which protect living people and corporations, to food.

In 1996, the connection between bovine spongiform encephalopathy and Creutzfeldt-Jakob disease was being discovered in the UK. Oprah Winfrey had a representative from the National Cattlemen's Beef Association, Gary Weber, and Howard Lyman, a former rancher and vegetarian advocate, on her show to discuss BSE and CJD. Lyman told Winfrey and the studio audience about the approximately 100,000 annual downer cows, many of whom are fed back to other cows in the form of rendered animal protein, and stated that were one of these cows to get into the domestic food supply, it could injure thousands. Winfrey replied, "Cows are herbivores. They shouldn't be eating other cows. . . . It has just stopped me cold from eating another burger" (Lyman 1998, 14).

A group of Texas cattlemen sued Winfrey and Lyman under the Texas Food Disparagement Act. Under the law, a person is liable if he knowingly gives information that states or implies a perishable food product is not safe for consumption by the public and that information is judged to be false according to reasonable and reliable scientific inquiry, facts, or data. In February 1998, a jury found in favor of Winfrey and Lyman.

Even though Winfrey and Lyman were not held liable, disparagement laws have the effect of quelling debate about the safety of food products. The influence of the thirteen states that have disparagement laws in practice extends to the whole country. Since much of the media is national, those that don't want to risk a lawsuit, or can't afford to risk a lawsuit, must tone down their remarks against particular foodstuffs.

Growth Hormones in Beef Cattle

Besides pesticides, there are many drugs used in agriculture that are controversial. These drugs, like pesticides, help increase yields. Since the 1950s, growth hormones have been used to increase meat production. Three naturally occurring hormones, estridiol, progesterone, and testosterone, and their synthetic equivalents, zeronol, acetate, and trebolone, are injected into calves' ears as time-release pellets. This implant under the skin causes the steers to gain an extra two to three pounds per week, and saves up to $80 per steer in production costs, because the steers gain more weight with the same amount of feed. Seventy-five percent of U.S. cattle are treated with hormones, but the European Union bans the practice and bans imported beef unless it is certified hormone-free (Jacobs 1999).

There is wide disagreement about whether the practice is safe. Hormone-like chemicals (DDT, PCBs, and dioxin) in large enough concentrations or at critical points in fetal development disrupt functioning of the natural hormones in both animal and human bodies. The U.S. government has been studying the endocrine disruptive effects of certain pesticides known as estrogenic (estrogen producing) and food contaminants known as xenoestrogens (substances that behave like estrogens), but they have not been studying hormones in meat. There has been escalating incidence of reproductive cancers in the United States since 1950. Breast cancer is up 55 percent, testicular cancer, 120 percent, and prostate cancer, 190 percent. No one knows the cause of these cancers, but even subtle shifts in quantities of hormones may contribute to the problem. Besides cancer, other estrogenic effects may include reduction in male fertility and early puberty. When exposed to higher than normal doses of estrogen through birth control pills or hormone replacement therapy in menopause, women experience somewhat higher risks of breast cancer and other tumors.

For many years, diethylstilbestrol (DES), a synthetic estrogen, was used to boost growth in cattle, sheep, and poultry. This same drug was used until the late 1960s to prevent miscarriage in humans. It was linked to a rare cancer in the daughters of treated mothers and was banned. It continued to be used in animals, however, until 1979 when the FDA pulled it from use for beef. Illegal use continued, and it was traced to baby food in Italy in 1980. Infant girls who consumed the tainted meat reportedly developed breasts and began menstruating. There were a number of prosecutions in the United States for illegal use. Partly because of the contamination of baby food and because of mad cow disease, the European Union outlawed the use of all hormones in meat and imposed a ban on imported meat treated with hormones in 1989 (Jacobs 1999).

The U.S. beef industry argues that the natural hormone levels in aging bulls and dairy cows used for beef in Europe can be many times higher than from steers treated with hormones. USDA officials note that the natural levels that occur in other animal foods, such as eggs, milk, and cheese, are substantially higher than the levels found in the tissue of treated animals. The USDA does not test for natural hormones and only sporadically tests for synthetic ones. A random USDA survey found as many as half of the steers had visible illegal, misplaced implants in muscle rather than under skin. This would result in very high local concentrations and elevated levels of hormones in muscle meats. Without regular testing it is difficult to know how high the hormone levels truly are.

The United States has put substantial pressure on Europe to accept its beef. The World Trade Organization appointed Codex Alimentarius Commission (the joint commission sponsored by WHO and FAO) to evaluate the safety of hormone-treated beef. The commission concluded that there is no scientific evidence to support the ban. However, according to Friends of the Earth, an environmental group, the commission is composed largely of representatives from multinational food manufacturers and pharmaceutical firms and the decisionmaking process denies reasonable access to the public (Friends of the Earth 1999).

The World Trade Organization concluded that the European Union ban was not based on risk assessment but rather was based on a belief in zero tolerance. The risk assessment process (described above) does have many unknowns and has the potential for bias. Large, long-term studies might show more definitively whether these hormones are safe.

Recombinant Bovine Growth Hormone

Similar controversy surrounds recombinant bovine growth hormone (rBGH), administered to dairy cattle to help them produce more milk. Developed by the Monsanto Corporation and marketed under the name Posilac, it has generated a lot of debate since it was approved by the FDA in 1993. The United States is the only major industrialized nation to approve rBGH. Health Canada, the food and drug regulatory arm of the Canadian government, rejected rBGH in early 1999 and stirred up more controversy in the process. They rejected the drug after careful review of the same data that were submitted to the U.S. FDA, finding that it did not meet standards for veterinary health and might pose food safety issues for humans.

The hormone is injected into the pituitary gland of dairy cows every two weeks because it can increase milk production by as much as 15 percent. Unfortunately, it increases the rate of mastitis (an infection of the udder) by 25 percent, increases the rate of infertility in cattle by 18 percent, and the rate of lameness by 50 percent (Hess 1999). Because the cows are sicker, they are dosed more heavily with antibiotics, which exacerbates the problem of antibiotic use in animals (see below). In order to produce more milk, the cows have to eat a higher-protein diet. Because corn is expensive, farmers often use feeds that include rendered animal protein. Ruminant to ruminant feeding is one of the factors that causes mad cow disease.

The mechanism by which rBGH works may also create dangerous hormones for people consuming the dairy products from treated cows. As a by-product, rBGH causes cows to produce more insulin growth factor 1 (IGF-1). IGF-1 is present in milk at higher levels in cows that take rBGH. IGF-1 causes cells to divide. Elevated levels have been associated with higher rates of breast, colon, ovarian, and prostate cancer and acromegaly, a disease characterized by abnormal enlargement of the nose, hands, feet, and chin. Monsanto claims that IGF-1 is killed during the pasteurization and digestion processes. However, other data discovered by Health Canada indicate it may survive ("Case Against Dairy" 1998).

The 90-day feeding study that was done by Monsanto to establish rBGH safety indicated that 20 to 30 percent of the rats fed a very high dose of rBGH developed antibodies to rBGH, which suggests that they had absorbed it into their bodies.

Monsanto scientists claimed that the rats had not absorbed it into their bloodstreams. Some male rats also developed cysts on their thyroids and increased mononuclear infiltration in the prostate (Bellow 1999). Although these studies do not in themselves indicate that rBGH will harm human health, they indicate that further long-term studies are needed to determine whether it is safe.

Many organizations have come out in favor of rBGH including the World Health Organization, the American Medical Association, and the American Dietetic Association ("FDA Charged" 1999). Some farmers like it, and others think it makes their cows sick. Estimates about use in the United States range from 8 to 30 percent of dairy cattle, but FDA rules do not permit a dairy to declare its milk rBGH free. Only milk labeled organic is assured to have no rBGH. Most milk is pooled so almost all the U.S. milk supply has at least traces of rBGH.

Antibiotics

Another class of drugs used for growth promotion is antibiotics. About 40 percent of all antibiotics produced are used in animal feed to speed growth and prevent diseases such as liver abscesses, foot rot, and enteritis. Agricultural industry groups attribute the relatively low prices of meat, milk, eggs, and cheese to the antibiotics that enhance growth. A 1981 USDA study found that antibiotics in feed save consumers about $3 billion per year (Ciment 1999). However, the use of antibiotics in animals has also been shown to increase bacterial resistance to antibiotics in humans.

When bacteria are confronted with an antibiotic, most of the bacteria die, but resistant bacteria survive. These bacteria reproduce, creating more resistant bacteria. The next time the antibiotic is given, more of the bacteria are likely to be resistant. Many scientists believe that giving low doses of antibiotics to animals on a regular basis breeds resistant bacteria. Additionally, bacteria are able to swap desirable traits even among different strains. For example, a salmonella bacterium living in the gut of a chicken could acquire the antibiotic resistance ability of a nearby E. coli bacterium.

In 1998, a strain of salmonella was found to be resistant to the newest class of antibiotics, fluoroquinolones, introduced in 1986. In the past, resistance has been fought with new classes of drugs that were coming out regularly. However, there are not currently any new classes of antibiotics that will be ready for approval in the near future. This has raised concern about the routine use of antibiotics in feed. On the recommendation of the World Health Organization, the European Union in 1998 banned the use of antibiotics that are used to treat humans to promote livestock growth (Ciment 1999). However, in the United States, six of the seventeen classes of antibiotics given to animals to promote growth are also given to treat illness in humans. Fluoroquinolones were approved for the treatment of chickens in 1995. A sharp rise in campylobacter fluoroquinolone resistance occurred in 1996, and in 1998 a Minnesota study found 10.2 percent of campylobacter cases were fluoroquinolone resistant (Grady 1999).

The FDA is currently revising its guidelines for approving new antibiotics for animals and for monitoring the effects of old ones. The Center for Science in the Public Interest led a campaign of forty-one organizations to require an outright ban on antibiotics in feed that are used to treat both humans and animals, similar to the European ban (Grady 1999).

Factory Farming

Antibiotics make factory farming possible. The discovery of the subtherapeutic use of antibiotics meant that animals could be confined in smaller spaces without contracting or spreading disease. There is a lot of disagreement about whether the animal products that come from factory farms are as safe as those that come from farms where the animals have more room. The animals suffer considerably more stress when they are placed in smaller spaces, do not have access to the outside, or cannot exercise. Some studies have shown that this stress leads to higher levels of disease. The process of factory farming is ultimately dangerous to human health because of contamination of groundwater and environmental destruction. It also negatively impacts food safety when manure too rich in nitrogen, trace minerals, heavy metals, and pathogens is used as fertilizer or runs off into rivers and contaminates fish.

Manure is the main by-product of factory farming. Approximately 316 billion pounds of dry weight animal wastes are produced in the United States each year (Michael Fox 1998). To put this number in perspective, total animal wastes are about forty times greater than human wastes (Wright 1999). Manure from large farms is handled in different ways. One problem is that large animal farms are often in different places than where crops are grown. The transportation cost of moving manure a thousand miles or more is prohibitive. Although some manure is put back into the soil, some is put into large lagoons where it decomposes anaerobically and generates greenhouse gases. Some of the manure is dried and fed to other animals. Cows are often fed dried chicken manure.

Small farms are often more environmentally friendly; they provide local uses for manure. However, ultimately, consumers must eat fewer animal products if we want to limit the environmental destruction caused by conventional agricultural practices.

Genetically Engineered Food

Drugs are one tool farmers use to improve yields and genetic engineering is another. Since ancient times, farmers have looked for ways to increase yields. Three-inch-long corncobs grown by Native Americans in Arizona have been replaced by the ten- and twelve-inch ears we see today. People saved seeds from successful plants, created hybrids, and enriched soil, among other methods of enhancing yields. Even since the 1960s, agriculture has become so much more efficient that it would take ten million more square miles of land to produce the same amount of crops we have today using the techniques of the 1960s. The latest method of improving productivity is genetic engineering, the transfer of DNA from organisms of one species into organisms of a different species (Shapiro 1999).

These DNA transfers can be used to make crops pest resistant and unaffected by herbicides, enhance nutritional qualities, or even create foods with medicinal qualities—such as bananas that inoculate the eaters against cholera, potatoes that prevent hepatitis, and tobacco and squash that prevent dental caries (Murray 1998). Genetically engineered corn seeds have a gene from the bacteria *Bacillus thuringiensis,* or Bt. This gene makes the corn plant resistant to the European corn borer, an insect that eats its way into the stalk and weakens the plant. Fields planted with the altered corn produce 6 to 8 percent greater yields on average (Belsie 1998).

Monsanto, the second largest agricultural engineering concern and the maker of the herbicide Round-Up, markets Round-Up-ready soybeans. These seeds are resistant to Round-Up, so the herbicide can be sprayed on the crops, killing the weeds and leaving the soybeans intact. The hope is that fewer herbicides can be used to control weeds, which would make the crops cheaper to grow and put fewer chemicals into the soil and groundwater. This could also mean fewer chemical residues on food.

Opponents of genetic engineering fear that these techniques will have only short-term benefits, and that "superweeds" will develop that will require the use of more toxic and greater quantities of herbicides. The Flavr Savr tomato, which was one of the earliest and most publicized genetically engineered products, was not a resounding commercial success and caused some to raise the issue of "faux freshness." If the tomato is engineered to have a long shelf life, will a consumer actually be purchasing an old tomato that looks fresh but has long since lost its nutritional value?

In the United States, the FDA ruled in May 1998 that food labeled organic could not be grown from genetically engineered seeds. In Europe, genetically engineered foods have met with great resistance. These foods are banned outright in Germany and Austria, corn only is allowed in France, and genetically modified foods must be labeled throughout the European Union. Some experts suggest that the British experience with mad cow disease has left the European community skittish of any changes that could affect the food supply.

So far scientific studies have not shown any problems with genetically engineered foods, but there may be long-term unforeseen consequences when we change our environment. In many other areas, changes in the ways food is grown and processed have created niches for harmful bacteria and viruses. Genetic engineering has much to offer in increasing the amount of food available to the world's expanding population, but the process should be carefully reviewed and tested to avoid creating new food risks and environmental catastrophes.

Functional Foods

Functional foods are foods that claim a health benefit because of something that was added to them. In the past, functional foods meant cereals fortified with additional vitamins or more recently calcium has been added to a variety of foods from orange juice to candy to snack bars. Now even more foods are being introduced with nutritional claims ranging from anticancer benefits, to cholesterol-lowering benefits, to mood- or memory-altering benefits. Kellogg's is making cereal with soy protein, Hains is making soup with St. John's wort (Somer 2000), BodyLogic is making snack bars with flaxseed, and Knudsen is making Simply Nutritious Ginkgo Alert, a soft drink.

Unfortunately, functional foods are not well regulated by the FDA. The FDA does not evaluate foods that are designed to improve general life conditions such as mood or mental sharpness. So including St. John's wort in foods does not require any testing for safety or efficacy. Even though the FDA examines claims for foods that target specific conditions like high cholesterol, it does not provide guidelines about appropriate doses or how ingredients might interact with a person's overall diet (Brown 2000).

Many products are not labeled with how much is included in the product, or what an appropriate quantity of the substance is. In the case of St. John's wort, Hains Creamy Split Pea Soup contains 98 milligrams of the herb. A standard dose is 1,000 to 2,000 milligrams taken daily for several weeks. Some experts advise buying regular products and taking supplements. This plan can be cheaper, too, as most functional foods cost more than their regular counterparts. Some functional foods are merely junk foods that have been fortified to make them seem healthy, like many of the energy bars currently on the market.

Side effects of herbs are often not considered, but some herbs do have negative side effects especially for individuals on medications for other conditions. People should also be very cautious about feeding functional foods to children. Herbs are essentially drugs that have had very little regulatory scrutiny, and children with smaller bodies and more vulnerable systems are at risk from untested products. Certain products, such as calcium-fortified candy, pose particular risks if children accidentally overdose on them (Somer 2000). Overall, functional foods should be evaluated carefully by consumers before purchase.

Food Additives

Before the FDA approves a new food additive or ingredient, its safety must be demonstrated. Animal feeding studies are performed to determine safety. Large doses are fed to a small number of rats to see whether they develop cancer or other diseases. Three ingredients, Olestra, aspartame (marketed as Equal or

NutraSweet), and hydrogenated fats have caused the most debate in recent years. However, many more additives are used, some of which are inert and some of which are unhealthy. Please see Chapter 4 for a complete summary of current food additives.

Olestra, a recently approved fat substitute, has been shown to diminish vitamin absorption and cause loose stools, diarrhea, and abdominal cramps in some individuals. The FDA decided the benefits of approving the product outweighed the negative effects but required special labeling for products containing Olestra.

Aspartame has caused adverse effects in some people, including dizziness, hallucinations, and headaches. However, controlled studies have yet to confirm these effects. There are also questions about the quality of the original cancer studies that were submitted to the FDA. Aspartame is consumed in such large quantities that further safety investigations should be pursued.

Hydrogenated oils are made when vegetable oil, a liquid, is treated with hydrogen to form a solid, shortening. This transformation has the effect of reducing polyunsaturated fats and increasing transfatty acids, which act like saturated fats and therefore promote heart disease. People at risk for heart disease should avoid hydrogenated fats and everyone else should consume them in moderation (Center for Science in the Public Interest 1999).

Irradiation

Just as science has brought us new food production techniques, it has also brought new food safety strategies such as irradiation. Irradiation is the process of subjecting food to electron beams or gamma rays to kill bacteria. The radiation damages the bacteria so that it cannot reproduce. By killing the bacteria, spoilage is also delayed. The amount of radiation is not enough to make the food radioactive, only to kill bacteria. Currently irradiation is used to sterilize medical supplies and cosmetics and a limited number of foods.

To irradiate food, the following process is used: (1) Metal carriers are loaded with boxes of food. (2) The carriers slide along an overhead monorail into a chamber containing radioactive cobalt, which is stored in a pool of water. (3) Hydraulic arms lift the cobalt out of the water pool exposing the boxes to gamma rays. Depending on the type of food, the duration of exposure varies. Frozen chicken takes as long as 20 minutes to irradiate; raw meat takes longer. (4) Once the food has been irradiated, the boxes slide out the opposite side and are loaded onto trucks for shipping to distributors or directly to restaurants and supermarkets (Gunther 1994).

Irradiation is the only way to kill *E. coli* O157:H7 besides heat. After the four deaths of children from *E. coli* O157:H7 that were traced to Jack in the Box restaurants in 1993, enthusiasm for irradiation grew and the USDA approved irradiation of beef in 1999. Irradiation raises the cost of meat by about five to ten cents per pound. Meat producers have been cautious about introducing irradiated beef because of the added cost and because it can darken meat and change the flavor enough to be noticeable. High-fat foods can develop a rancid smell. Irradiated food must be marked with the radura symbol or it must say "irradiated" on the food label (Rothstein 1998).

The marketing departments of grocery and meat trade organizations have found that considerable education of consumers is needed before they will accept irradiation, and it is likely that a new name for the process will be adopted, such as cold pasteurization or electronic, or ionizing, pasteurization. Market demand will have to be seen in order for investment to be made in the large-scale facilities that would be needed to process large quantities of food.

Besides increased cost and potential reduction of food taste, there are several drawbacks to irradiation. When the food is bombarded with radiation, some of the electrons are freed and attach to other atoms forming new compounds, some of which are harmful like benzene and formaldehyde. Free radicals called unidentified radiolytic particles are also present. No one knows exactly what effect these particles might have. Many generations of rats have been fed irradiated food without any ill effects. However, no feeding studies have been done in which these particles are concentrated and fed at high doses to animals, giving them a dose that is one hundred times the normal. This is the standard method of testing for carcinogenic properties.

There is also significant vitamin loss from irradiation. Vitamins A, B(1), B(3), B(6), B(12), C, E, and K, and folic acid are affected. In some foods, as little as 10 percent of the vitamins are destroyed, but in others it can be as high as 50 percent. If irradiated foods become a major part of people's diets, overall nutritional quality will suffer. And while irradiation kills most bacteria, it does not affect viruses, and any bacteria that gets onto food after treatment suddenly has a food supply without any competitors. This creates the potential for very toxic food. Some groups, such as Food and Water, an organization devoted to food purity issues, also believe that irradiation could allow the causes of meat contamination to flourish because producers would not be forced to clean up filthy and sloppy processing facilities when they could simply irradiate fecal-contaminated meat products that should be discarded (Nicols Fox 1998).

Hazard Analysis and Critical Control Points

Many people believe that Hazard Analysis and Critical Control Points techniques are superior to irradiation. HACCP is a method of improving food safety developed by Pillsbury for NASA in the late 1950s (Lewis 1998). HACCP requires determining the food safety hazards that are likely to occur and, by using that knowledge, establishing procedures at critical points to ensure safety. HACCP can be applied at any point in the food cycle from field to fork. The steps, which are modified for each setting, include analyzing the setting for potential problem areas, examining inputs to the system such as suppliers, determining prevention and control measures, taking action when criteria aren't met, and establishing and maintaining record-keeping procedures. Some settings require microbial testing for bacteria.

HACCP is very adaptable to different settings. A rangeland watershed in Alameda County, California, is being managed with HACCP techniques to guard against the parasite cryptosporidium and other potential pathogens. The techniques used in this setting include managing stocking rates of cattle to maintain enough vegetative cover, excluding calves from areas directly adjacent to the reservoirs, locating water and supplemental feed away from stream channels, maintaining herd health programs, and implementing a feral pig control program. Testing water regularly ensures the success of the program and will help identify additional control points and management measures ("Development and Use" 1998).

A farm in Fresno County, California, that supplies Odwalla, a fresh juice producer, has implemented HACCP in the fields. All field bins are washed prior to use; bins are never put on the ground; workers wash their hands routinely throughout the day; each worker must be certified healthy; all water sources are tested regularly; field toilets are cleaned daily; use of toilets is managed and mandated; and third-party audits are posted on the Internet (McAFee 1998).

In a manufacturing plant, HACCP is very compatible with good manufacturing practices (GMPs), which include proper sanitation procedures. HACCP takes GMPs a step further by looking at other potential problem areas. For example, a juice producer following GMPs emphasizes fruit washing, plant cleanliness, and strict adherence to sanitary policies and procedures. To implement HACCP, the plant adds pasteurization to some products, ensures a cold-chain by making sure the product always stays cold, and performs microbial testing to make sure the procedures are working. Following these procedures could drastically reduce the 16,000 to 48,000 annual illnesses the FDA attributes to juice consumption (Rice 1998).

The Jack in the Box restaurant chain has developed HACCP to a highly refined system since the 1993 *E. coli* outbreak that resulted from tainted meat from one of its suppliers. Now the restaurant chain does extensive microbial testing, testing the ground beef off the production line every 15 minutes. The distribution company has installed time and temperature recording boxes that record the temperature in the delivery trucks to ensure that the beef is always stored at the proper temperature (Steinauer 1997).

In a retail establishment, recipes and procedures must be revised to make food as safe as possible. This could mean changing a recipe to ensure that foods that are added raw are chopped in a separate place from items that are chopped before cooking. Suppliers are carefully examined, food is maintained at the proper temperature, and the length of time foods are left out is closely monitored. For example, a policy that unsold chicken nuggets will be thrown out every half hour might be implemented with a timer that beeps on the half hour. Employees might have to initial a log stating that they had disposed of unsold food.

HACCP has been mandatory for the low-acid canned food industry and went into effect for domestic and imported seafood processing in 1997. Meat and poultry processors had to implement HACCP plans in January 2000. There is some evidence that

HACCP is working. A 1999 study showed ground beef samples tested positive for salmonella 7.5 percent of the time prior to HACCP and 4.3 percent of the time after implementation. Similarly, salmonella in chickens has dropped from 20 percent to 10.7 percent, and in pork from 8.7 percent to 6.2 percent ("Reflects HACCP 'Payoff'" 1999).

These results are very encouraging, but safe food practices must become part of a company's or institution's culture in order to be followed. Some companies have had good results by offering incentives for safe practices, making safe food procedures an important part of performance evaluations, ensuring that managers model safe food behaviors, and instituting procedures that require an employee to keep records or sign records that are checked. Documentation has traditionally not been a part of food service workers' jobs, and some companies have gone to automated processes to make the job easier. McDonald's Corporation has installed a hygiene system, which monitors hand washing. Before an employee washes his hands, he punches in his personal ID code. The system tracks how often and how long an employee spends washing his hands (Steinauer 1997).

New Food Safety Techniques

Besides technologies that reinforce commonsense hygiene practices, there are several new techniques and technologies that show promise. One such technique is high-pressure processing. At the National Center for Food Safety and Technology, engineers have developed a high-pressure system that delivers 90,000 pounds of pressure. The pressure is enough to kill bacteria, although not viruses. It is appropriate for homogenized products such as guacamole.

Other technologies include low-temperature pasteurization using a pulsed electric field that could be used for orange juice. This would allow orange juice to be pasteurized at 86 degrees instead of 200 degrees F and would thus improve the flavor. Steam pasteurization of meat carcasses can kill bacteria such as *E. coli*. The carcass is steamed quickly, so as not to cook the meat. A manufacturer in the Midwest recently began marketing eggs that had been pasteurized in their shells at low heat. These eggs are now safe for mayonnaise, eggnog, and being served sunny-side up (Springen 1998).

Other technologies work to prevent contamination before it happens. A drug spray, called PreEmpt, was recently approved by the FDA. It is sprayed on chicks, and contains twenty-nine living, nontoxic bacteria that invade the chicks' intestines, crowding out more harmful bacteria such as campylobacter, salmonella, listeria, and *E. coli* O157:H7. The manufacturer, MSBioscience, is currently at work on similar sprays for cattle and swine (Hunter 1999).

Protecting Yourself from Food Poisoning

Although new technologies can help overall food safety, there are many things individuals can do to protect themselves from illness. These steps won't completely eliminate problems, but they will minimize hazards.

1. Wash your hands regularly and especially after using the toilet, before preparing food, and after handling raw meat.
2. Wash vegetables and fruits before eating. Discard the outside leaves of lettuce.
3. Use separate cutting boards and utensils for raw meat. Raw meat should not come in contact with any foods that will be eaten raw. If you place meat on a plate to carry it out to a grill, use a clean plate for the cooked meat.
4. Sponges should be washed in the dishwasher daily and replaced often.
5. Immune compromised people should avoid packaged meats and prepared salads.
6. Keep cold foods cold, and hot foods hot. Leftovers should be stored promptly and reheated thoroughly before eating. Leftovers should be used within three to four days.
7. If food is spoiled, no amount of reheating or chilling will compensate. If food has been left out too long, it should be discarded.
8. Avoid eating raw eggs. This includes uncooked cookie dough and cake batters. In place of raw eggs, pasteurized eggs, such as EggBeaters, can be used.

9. Hamburger should be thoroughly cooked before eating. Since oxidation turns meat brown, verify that the meat is cooked by checking with a meat thermometer. It should read 160 degrees F.

References

Altekruse, Sean F., et al. "Campylobacter Jejuni—An Emerging Foodborne Pathogen." *Emerging Infectious Diseases* 5, no. 1 (January–February 1999): 28–35.

Antin, Angel. "Dealing with Deadly Bacteria." *Public Relations Tactics* 5, no. 3 (March 1998): 1–3.

Bellow, Daniel. "Vermont: The Pure Food State: How Farmers and Citizens Fought the Use of Monsanto's Hormone for Cows." *The Nation* 268, no. 9 (March 8, 1999): 18–21.

Belsie, Laurent. "Altered Seeds: Biotech Farming." *Christian Science Monitor.* July 30, 1998. B1.

Blakeslee, Sandra. "British Mad Cow Disease Toll Rises, but the Cause Is Unclear." *New York Times.* March 19, 1999. A8.

Bonner, John. "Antibiotics in Animal Nutrition." *New Scientist* 153, no. 2065 (January 18, 1997): 24–27.

Borzelleca, Joseph. "Food-Borne Health Risks: Food Additives, Pesticides, and Microbes." In *Nutrition Policy in Public Health,* ed. Felix Bronner. New York: Springer, 1997.

Brown, Kathryn. "Food with Attitude." *Discover* 21, no. 3 (March 2000): 31–32.

"Case Against Dairy." *Vegetarian Times*, no. 254 (October 1998): 90–92.

Center for Science in the Public Interest. "Chemical Cuisine: CSPI's Guide to Food Additives." http://www.cspinet.org/reports/chemcuisine.htm. April 18, 1999.

Ciment, James. "FDA Proposes Measuring Antibiotics in Feed." *British Medical Journal* 318, no. 7187 (March 27, 1999): 829.

Couzin, Jennifer. "Cattle Diet Linked to Bacterial Growth." *Science* 281, no. 5383 (September 11, 1998): 578–1579.

"Cull Maff." *The Economist* 349, no. 8096 (November 28, 1998): 61.

DeNoon, Daniel, and Keith Key. "Salmonella and Campylobacter Illnesses on the Decline." *Health Letter on the CDC* (March 29–April 5, 1999): 3–4.

"Development and Use of a HACCP Program to Protect Water Quality in a Rangeland Watershed." *Journal of Soil and Water Conservation* 53, no. 2 (Second Quarter 1998): 173.

Dickerson, Marla. "Private Health Auditors Are Serving Diners, Restaurants." *Los Angeles Times.* April 7, 1999. C1, C6.

Efron, Sonni. "Japanese Choke on American Biofood." *Los Angeles Times.* March 14, 1999. A1, A8–9.

"FDA Charged with Ignoring Bgh Hazards." *Chemical Market Reporter* 255, no. 1 (January 4, 1999): 6–7.

Fox, Michael. "Manure, Minerals, and Methane: How Factory Farms Threaten the Environment." *The Animals Agenda* 18, no. 3 (May/June 1998): 30–32.

Fox, Nicols. "Irradiation: Will It Make Our Food Safe to Eat?" *Vegetarian Times*, no. 247 (March 1998): 74–80.

Fox, Nicols. *Spoiled: The Dangerous Truth About a Food Chain Gone Haywire.* New York: Basic Books, 1997.

Freeman, Laurie. "'Irradiation' Designation May Finally Become a Sales Pitch." *Marketing News* 32, no. 19 (September 14, 1998): 1–3.

Friends of the Earth. "WTO Scorecard: The Beef Hormones Case: Steer on Steroids." http://www.foe.org/international/trade/wto/cows.htm. April 25, 1999.

Giamalva, John N., et al. "Dieticians Employed by Health Care Facilities Preferred HACCP System over Irradiation or Chemical Rinses for Reducing Risk of Foodborne Disease." *Journal of the American Dietetic Association* 98, no. 8 (August 1998): 885–888.

Grady, Denise. " A Move to Limit Antibiotic Use in Animal Feed." *New York Times.* March 8, 1999. A1, A13.

Graebner, Lynn. "UCD Sheds New Light on Anti-Bacteria Technology." *Sacramento Business Journal* 15, no. 38 (December 4, 1998): 1.

Green, Emily. "Britain Details the Start of Its 'Mad Cow' Outbreak." *New York Times.* January 26, 1999. F2.

Gunther, Judith Anne. "The Food Zappers." *Popular Science* 244, no. 1 (January 1994): 72–78.

Hess, Glenn. "Canada Rejects Bovine Growth Hormone; Monsanto Vows to Appeal the Decision." *Chemical Market Reporter* 255, no. 4 (January 25, 1999): 1–2.

Hingley, Audrey. "Rallying the Troops to Fight Food-Borne Illness." *FDA Consumer* 31, no. 7 (November–December 1997): 7–9.

Hunter, Beatrice Trum. "Innovative Safety Techniques." *Consumers' Research Magazine* 82, no. 2 (February 1999): 8–9.

Jacobs, Paul. "U.S., Europe Lock Horns in Beef Hormone Debate." *Los Angeles Times.* April 9, 1999. A1, A10.

Jaykus, Lee-Ann. "Epidemiology and Detection as Options for Control of Viral and Parasitic Foodborne Disease." *Emerging Infectious Disease* 3 (October–December 1997): 529–540.

Key, Sandra W., ed. "E. Coli Infections Appear to Be Increasing." *Health Letter on the CDC.* June 9, 1997. 7–8.

Key, Sandra W., ed. "E. Coli O157:H7: Difficult to Remove from the Food Supply." *Disease Weekly Plus.* October 20, 1997. 18–19.

Key, Sandra W., ed. "Illnesses Linked to Alfalfa Sprouts." *World Disease Weekly Plus.* March 8, 1999. 16–7.

Kluger, Jeffrey. "Anatomy of an Outbreak." *Time* 142, no. 5 (August 3, 1998): 56–62.

Koutkia, Polyxeni, et al. "Enterohemorrhagic Escherichia Coli O157:H7—An Emerging Pathogen." *American Family Physician* 56, no. 3 (September 1, 1997): 853–856.

Kurtzweil, Paula. "Safer Eggs: Laying the Groundwork." *FDA Consumer* 32, no. 5 (September–October 1998): 10–15.

Lammerding, Anna M., and Greg M. Paoli. "Quantitative Risk Assessment: An Emerging Tool for Emerging Foodborne Pathogens." *Emerging Infectious Disease* 3, no. 4 (October–December 1997): 483–487.

Lewis, Len. "Retail Culinary: Hassling with HACCP." *Progressive Grocer* 77, no. 5 (May 1998): 165–169.

Licking, Ellen, and John Carey. "How to Head Off the Next Tainted-Food Disaster." *Business Week,* no. 3618 (March 1, 1999): 34.

Lovett, Richard A. "Training a Molecular Gun on Killer E. Coli." *Science* 282, no. 5393 (November 20, 1998): 1404.

Lyman, Howard, and Glen Merzer. *Mad Cowboy: Plain Truth from the Cattle Rancher Who Won't Eat Meat.* New York: Scribner, 1998.

Margaronis, Maria. "Greenwashed." *The Nation* 267, no. 12 (October 19, 1998): 10.

Maugh, Thomas H. "Gene Discovery May Lead to New Vaccines." *Los Angeles Times.* May 7, 1999. A3.

McAFee, Mark. "Valley Grown Food Safety Procedures Recognized Nationally." *The Business Journal Serving Fresno and the Central San Joaquin Valley,* no. 322394 (December 14, 1998): 27.

McCarthy, Michael. "E. Coli O157:H7 Outbreak Traced to Apple Juice." *Lancet* 348, no. 9037 (November 9, 1996): 1299.

McConnell, Harvey. "Antibiotics and Superbugs." *Futurist* 33, no. 2 (February 1999): 9.

McDermott, Karen Govel. "Making HACCP Work." *Nation's Restaurant News* 32, no. 28 (July 13, 1998): 51.

McGraw, Linda. "Battling Food-Poisoning Bacteria." *Agricultural Research* 47, no. 2 (February 1999): 12–13.

Motavalli, Jim. "A Brave New World: Genetic Engineering, Rbgh, and Mad Cow Disease." *E. Magazine: The Environmental Magazine* (July 1996).

Murray, Joan. "What Happened to Flavr Savr?" *Food Service Director* 11, no. 11 (November 15, 1998): 98.

Pace, Janet. "Something You Ate?" *Chatelaine* 71, no. 7 (July 1998): 36–42.

Parseghian, Pam. "Cook Up Safety Precautions When Serving Raw Fish." *Nation's Restaurant News* 31, no. 22 (June 2, 1997): 33.

Puzo, Daniel. "3 Out of 5 Chickens in U.S. Test Found to Have Salmonella." *Los Angeles Times.* May 4, 1990. A1.

"Reflects HACCP 'Payoff': USDA Sees Food Safety Gains." *Food Service Director.* March 15, 1999.

Rice, Judy. "HACCP and GMPs Spell Greater S-A-F-E-T-Y for Fresh Juice Industry." *Beverage Industry* 89, no. 6 (June 1998): 44–45.

Riell, Howard. "The Real Test for HACCP: 'Making Food-Safety Part of the Culture.'" *Food Service Director* 11, no. 2 (February 15, 1998): 144.

Rothstein, Linda. "An Idea Whose Time Has Come—and Gone?" *The Bulletin of the Atomic Scientists* 54, no. 4 (July–August 1998): 7–8.

Rubinstein, Ed. "Automated Tools Make HACCP Less Burdensome for Operators." *Nation's Restaurant News* 32, no. 47 (November 23, 1998): 18–19.

Rubinstein, Ed. "The 'Beefs' over Food Irradiation Begin to Simmer." *Nation's Restaurant News* 32, no. 20 (May 18, 1998): 71–72.

Schardt, David. "Cow Disease Still Mad." *Nutrition Action Health Letter* 26, no. 3 (April 1999): 10.

Schnittker, John. "An Agricultural Revolution with Implications for Sustainability." *Choices: The Magazine of Food, Farm, and Resource Issues* 13, no. 3 (Fourth Quarter 1998): 1.

Schumann, Michael S., et al. *Food Safety Law.* New York: Van Nostrand Reinhold, 1997.

Shapiro, Robert. "How Genetic Engineering Will Save Our Planet." *Futurist* 33, no. 4 (April 1999): 28–29.

Shell, Ellen Ruppel. "Could Mad-Cow Disease Happen Here?" *Atlantic Monthly* 282, no. 3 (September 1998): 92–103.

Sicakyuz, Achrene. "France's *Fromage Fatale.*" *Los Angeles Times.* April 28, 1999. H1-H2.

Smith, Gar. "Did Monsanto Fake Science?" *Earth Island Journal* 14, no. 1 (Winter–Spring 1999): 27.

Somer, Elizabeth. "Waiter, There's St. John's Wort in My Soup." *Prevention* 52, no. 2 (February 2000): 140–145.

Spake, Amanda. "Deadly Hot Dogs and Ham." *U.S. News & World Report* (February 22, 1999): 62.

Springen, Karen. "Safer Food for a Tastier Millennium." *Newsweek* 132, no. 13 (September 28, 1998): 14.

Steinauer, Joan. "Natural Born Killers." *Incentive* 171, no. 10 (November 1997): 24–29.

United States Food and Drug Administration. *Foodborne Pathogenic Microorganisms and Natural Toxins Handbook.* http://vm.cfsan.fda.gov/~dms/fc-toc.html. May 25, 1999.

Waltner-Toews, David. *Food, Sex and Salmonella: The Risks of Environmental Intimacy.* Toronto: NC Press, 1992.

Waverly, Ken S. "Irradiation and Mad Cow Disease: What! Me Worry?" *Countryside and Small Stock Journal* 82, no. 4 (July–August 1998): 105.

World Health Organization. "Food Safety: An Essential Public Health Issue for the New Millennium." http://www.who.int/fsf. 1999.

Wright, Andrew. "A Foul Mess: EPA Takes Aim at Factory Farms, the Number One Water Polluter in U.S." *Engineering News Record* 243, no. 14 (October 4, 1999): 26–30.

Wright, Karen. "Raspberries in America." *Discover the World of Science* 18, no. 1 (January 1997): 88.

2

Chronology

Ancient times	Ancient Greek and Roman laws prohibit adulteration or addition of impurities to wine.
1206	King John of England prohibits adulteration of bread.
1266	English law enacted that prohibits the practices of short-weighting customers and selling unsound meat.
1822	Frederick C. Marcus, a German chemist living in London, publishes *A Treatise on Adulteration of Food and Culinary Poisons.* A pirated version appears in the United States. Marcus reveals that many common foodstuffs are adulterated.
1872	England enacts Adulteration of Food or Drink Act with stiff penalties for violations, including six months' hard labor for the second offense. This act is not modernized until 1955, when the Food and Drug Act is passed.
1880s	Women's groups around the United States begin to organize for pure food, drink, and drugs. In 1884, fifteen Beekman Hill women declare war on New York City's slaughterhouse district, a tangle of fifty-five broken-down wooden sheds that reek with filth from accumulated refuse and slaughter. Through the women's persistence, lawsuits, and negotiations with

1880s   the Health Department, the slaughterhouses are
(*cont.*)   cleaned up in the early 1890s. Also in 1884, the
           Women's Christian Temperance Union teaches classes
           to delegates at its national convention in Battle Creek,
           Michigan, on how to rid U.S. homes of dangerous and
           adulterated food, drink, and drugs.

1883   U.S. Tea Act of 1883 attempts to prevent sale of adul-
           terated teas. The law proves to be useless because it
           sets no standards and no method of enforcement.

1890   First U.S. food inspection law is enacted. Although
           this act benefits consumers, it is established by mer-
           chants trying to convince foreign companies that U.S.
           foods are safe.

1897   Tea Importation Act of 1897 makes it illegal to import
           tea that is inferior in purity, quality, and fitness for
           consumption.

1902   Harvey Wiley, director of the Bureau of Chemistry,
           starts a "poison squad" to test common food additives.
           Volunteer testers are fed a carefully controlled diet to
           test for adverse effects. One at a time, a different addi-
           tive is incorporated into the diet in high quantities.

1906   *The Jungle* by Upton Sinclair is published. It details the
           unsanitary practices of the meatpacking industry. Six
           months after publication, the Pure Food and Drug Bill
           and the Beef Inspection Bill are passed.

           Pure Food and Drug Law and Food and Drug Acts of
           1906, administered by the U.S. Bureau of Chemistry,
           provide the basic legal and institutional frameworks
           for our current food safety laws. These laws prohibit
           the shipment in interstate commerce of foods that are
           adulterated by any of several definitions, including
           food that is spoiled, contaminated with filth, derived
           from diseased animals, or containing unsafe sub-
           stances.

Federal Meat Inspection Act is administered by the USDA since its inception. Meat requires continuous, on-site factory inspection by government inspectors using sight, smell, and touch to detect unsafe meat.

1910   Insecticide Act marks the federal government's first attempt to regulate pesticides.

1913   Gould Amendment of the Food and Drug Acts requires that net contents must be stated on the label.

1914   The Federal Trade Commission Act establishes Federal Trade Commission and empowers it to monitor food advertising.

1920s   French scientists discover irradiation preserves food.

1923   Filled Milk Act prohibits the sale of milk to which fats or oils, other than milk fats, have been added.

1927   Federal Milk Importation Act establishes regulations on importation of milk and cream into the United States to protect public health.

1930   USDA Bureau of Chemistry is renamed Food and Drug Administration (FDA).

1938   Federal Food, Drug and Cosmetic Act gives the FDA authority to perform plant inspections, to establish standards of identity for individual food products, and to certify colors (colors are divided into categories based on whether they can be used in food, drugs, and cosmetics [F, D, and C colors]; or just drugs and cosmetics; or cosmetics only). The act also grants the FDA the right to seek injunctions in federal court against violators of the law.

1939   Swiss chemist Paul Muller recognizes the value of dichlorodiphenyl-trichloroethane (DDT) as a potent nerve poison that will work on insects, ushering in a new era in agricultural pesticides. DDT is successfully

1939 (cont.)	used during World War II to kill malaria-causing insects. Muller wins the Nobel Prize for his work in 1948, but realizes the harm DDT can do to the environment, wildlife, and humans because of its persistence.
1940s	U.S. Army begins testing irradiation of common foods.
1940	FDA becomes part of the U.S. Federal Security Agency.
1944	Public Health Service Act gives the FDA authority over vaccines and serums and is allowed to inspect restaurants and travel facilities.
1947	Federal Insecticide, Fungicide, and Rodenticide Act (FIFRA) establishes criteria used to evaluate the safety of pesticides. Pesticides must now be licensed, proven effective, and hazards must be accurately labeled. This law is primarily a labeling law and only applies to pesticides used to produce goods sold in interstate commerce.
1949	Dr. Thomas Jukes, then director of nutrition and physiology research at Lederle's Pharmaceutical Company, discovers that animals fed small doses of antibiotics gain weight faster.
Early 1950s	Farmers begin feeding livestock antibiotics subtherapeutically to prevent and treat subclinical disease (diseases that don't cause evident symptoms, but are nonetheless taxing to the animal) and to promote growth. By 1954, U.S. farmers are using 245 tons of antibiotics each year in livestock feed.
1953	FDA becomes a separate entity in the Department of Health, Education, and Welfare. This department is later renamed the Department of Health and Human Services.

1954   Miller Amendment to the Federal Food, Drug, and Cosmetic Act allows the FDA to establish tolerances for "economic poisons," or pesticides, on agricultural products like fruit, vegetables, and grains.

1957   Poultry Products Inspection Act of 1957 requires that poultry products be wholesome, unadulterated, properly marked, labeled, and packaged. Poultry is now subject to the same inspection criteria as beef; it must be continuously monitored and inspected in the factory.

The first commercial use of irradiation takes place in Stuttgart, Germany, where the process is used to preserve spices.

1958   Food Additives Amendment to the FDCA empowers the FDA to prohibit additives to food that have not been adequately tested to establish safety. In effect the FDA also has premarket review and approval authority over chemical additives in foods. This amendment includes the Delaney Clause (after the congressman responsible for its inclusion), which states that no additive will be deemed safe if any quantity of the additive is found to cause cancer in humans or any animal species. As part of this amendment, irradiation is regulated as a food additive rather than a preservation process. Therefore, irradiation must meet a higher standard of proof before it will be declared safe.

Humane Slaughter Act requires cattle and pigs to be rendered senseless to pain before being shackled, hoisted, thrown, cast, or cut. The act only applies to animals whose meat is sold to the federal government, but in practice the act is applied in all commercial plants.

1959   Germany passes a law banning irradiation, and the machine used to process spices in Stuttgart (see 1957) is dismantled.

1960s   Pillsbury Corporation, under contract from NASA, develops Hazard Analysis and Critical Control Points (HACCP) to protect the astronauts from foodborne illness. HACCP as originally conceived by Pillsbury includes (1) identification and assessment of hazards associated with growing and harvesting to marketing and preparation; (2) determination of the critical control points to control any identifiable hazard; and (3) establishment of systems to monitor critical control points.

Scientists working at Keio University's School of Medicine in Japan including Tsutomo Watanabe and Stuart Levy discover that antibiotic drug resistance is a transferable trait between different strains of bacteria. For example, a strain of salmonella that is resistant to penicillin can pass on this resistance to a strain of campylobacter.

1960   Color Additives Amendment makes pretesting requirements uniform. Previously the FDA could not set limits on the amounts of color that could be used. This act requires the FDA to consider the probable consumption levels of the color, cumulative effects, substances formed as a result of consumption of the color, safety factors, and potential carcinogenicity.

1961   The Food and Agriculture Organization and the World Health Organization, both agencies of the United Nations, establish the Codex Alimentarius Commission to set standards, including technical specifications and good manufacturing practices. The purpose of the standards is to facilitate trade between nations and ensure safe food.

1962   *Silent Spring* by Rachel Carson is published. Carson, a marine biologist, describes the environmental damage caused by DDT in the environment.

1963   Irradiation is approved by the FDA to control insects in wheat and wheat powder.

1964   FDA approves irradiation to extend the shelf life of white potatoes.

1966   Fair Packaging and Labeling Act requires that all labels contain the same basic information, including common or usual name of product, name and address of manufacturer, ingredients in order of weight, net weight, and a statement that the product contains artificial color or flavor, if any.

1967   Wholesome Meat Act is a complete revision of the 1906 act. Meat must be wholesome, unadulterated, properly marked, labeled, and packaged. All cattle, sheep, swine, and goats must be inspected prior to slaughter. Previous legislation applied to meat sold in interstate commerce only. Now state inspection standards must be at least equal to federal standards. Additionally, the Department of Agriculture has the power to seize unsafe meat and federal regulators may examine company records.

1968   Poultry Products Act extends federal poultry inspection standards to poultry produced and sold within the same state. In 1968 87 percent of poultry was federally inspected. This act extends inspection to the remaining 13 percent.

1970s   NASA adopts irradiation to sterilize food for astronauts.

1970   Egg Products Inspection Act requires that eggs be wholesome, not adulterated, and properly labeled and packaged. Egg products must be continuously monitored and inspected in the factory.

        The International Atomic Energy Agency (IAEA), Food and Agriculture Organization (FAO), World Health Organization (WHO), and the Organization for Economic Cooperation and Development (OECD) create the International Project in the Field of Food

1970
(cont.)

Irradiation to sponsor a worldwide research program on the wholesomeness of irradiated foods.

The Environmental Protection Agency is created (EPA). Regulation of pesticides is transferred from the U.S. Department of Agriculture (USDA) to the new agency.

Cyclamate, a type of artificial sweetener, is banned by the FDA. At the time, it was thought to cause bladder cancer and damage to the testes. Current research suggests that it does not cause cancer directly, but increases the potency of other carcinogens.

1971

The Hazard Analysis and Critical Control Points concept is presented to the public for the first time at the 1971 National Conference on Food Protection.

1972

Federal Environmental Pesticide Control Act revises FIFRA. All pesticides must now be registered with the Environmental Protection Agency. This includes pesticides that were previously excluded because they were not used on foodstuffs sold across state lines. This legislation makes it easier to ban hazardous pesticides and imposes penalties for improper use. The law divides pesticides into two categories: general use and restricted use. Restricted use pesticides must be clearly labeled and may only be used by certified applicators.

DDT is banned in the United States except for use in extreme health emergencies.

1973

About one ton of polybrominated biphenyl (PBB), a closely related but much more toxic chemical than polychlorinated biphenyl (PCB), is mistakenly added to cattle feed in Michigan. It is estimated that virtually all the citizens of Michigan and some of the citizens of other states consumed the substance either in dairy products or meat.

1974   In the Safe Drinking Water Act, the EPA is directed to establish national standards setting the maximum allowable levels for certain chemical and bacteriological pollutants for water systems serving more than twenty-five customers.

1976   Red dyes number one and two are banned by the FDA. Red dye number one is found to cause liver cancer, and red dye number two is found to be a possible carcinogen.

1977   The FDA bans saccharin because many animal studies show that it causes cancer of the bladder. Other studies show it may also cause other cancers. In 1977 saccharin is the primary sweetener in diet soft drinks and a number of other artificially sweetened products, and the U.S. public is outraged at the ban. However, before the ban can take effect, Congress intervenes. Saccharin continues to be available but must carry a warning notice. An interesting consequence of these actions is a weakening of public support for the Delaney clause, which does not permit cancer-causing food additives in any amount.

1979   Diethylstilbestrol (DES) is banned for use in cattle. Other growth hormones may still be used.

1980   As a result of the research started in 1970, the Joint Food and Agriculture Organization/World Health Organization/International Atomic Energy Agency Expert Committee on the Wholesomeness of Irradiated Foods concludes that the irradiation of any food commodity up to an overall dose of 10 kilograys (kGy) presents no toxicological hazard. Therefore, toxicological testing of foods so treated is no longer required.

National Academy of Sciences issues a report entitled, "The Effects on Human Health of Subtherapeutic Use of Antibiotics in Animal Feed." The report states that almost half of the antibiotics manufactured in the

1980 (cont.)	United States are fed to animals, but the academy is unable to determine from existing research whether antibiotics in animal feed harm human health.
1981	Aspartame, the artificial sweetener marketed under the names NutraSweet and Equal, is approved by the FDA for use in drinks, mixes, desserts, and cold cereals. It is 200 times sweeter than sugar, and one teaspoon has one-tenth of a calorie.
1983	The FDA approves irradiation for spices and dry vegetable seasonings to kill insects and bacteria.
1984	U.S. Environmental Protection Agency asks the National Academy of Sciences to explore the level of protection that law and regulation provide against cancer risks from pesticide residues in food. The academy forms the Delaney Committee to address this question.
1985	The largest ever outbreak of salmonella poisoning occurs in Illinois. The source is traced to a milk plant where one day's output was incorrectly pasteurized. Over 200,000 people are affected and four people die.

Nearly one thousand people in several western states and Canada are poisoned by pesticide residues from the pesticide Temik in watermelons. Symptoms included nausea, vomiting, blurred vision, and muscle weakness. Some become gravely ill and suffer grand mal seizures and cardiac irregularities. At least two stillbirths result from the poisoning.

A subcommittee of the Food Protection Committee of the National Academy of Sciences issues a report on microbiological criteria strongly endorsing HACCP. The report recommends that both regulators and industry use HACCP because it is the most effective and efficient means of ensuring the safety of our food supply.

The FDA approves low-dose irradiation to control trichinella in pork.

1986   First cases of bovine spongiform encephalopathy (BSE) are confirmed in Britain. The disease is nick-named "mad cow disease" because the cows stagger around as if drunk, become belligerent, and die.

FDA approves irradiation for fruits and vegetables. It is used both to control insects and to slow the ripening of fruits and vegetables.

1987   National Academy of Sciences issues a report on pesticides entitled "Regulating Pesticides: The Delaney Paradox." The Delaney Committee finds that nearly all registrations for pesticide use on food crops are set using a risk benefit balancing standard contained within the Federal Insecticide, Fungicide, and Rodenticide Act. Using this standard does not protect the public from significant health risk. The higher Delaney standard, which requires that strict limits be placed on pesticides suspected of inducing cancer, is used in only 3 percent of cases. Using these data, it is estimated that there will be an additional 1 million cancer cases over a seventy-year period.

1988   Pesticide Monitoring and Improvements Act requires a computerized monitoring system for the FDA to record, summarize, and evaluate results of its program for monitoring food products for pesticide residues.

An expert scientific advisory panel to the secretaries of Agriculture, Commerce, Defense, and Health and Human Services, the National Advisory Committee on Microbiological Criteria for Foods (NACMCF), is convened. Part of the mission of NACMCF is to promote adoption of HACCP principles.

The British government appoints a committee to assess any possible risk to human health from BSE in

1988   cattle. At the committee's recommendation, a ban is
(cont.)   placed on feeding animal-derived protein to rumi-
            nants like cattle, and farmers must report suspected
            cases of BSE. Over two thousand confirmed cases of
            BSE are reported in 1988.

1989   CBS broadcasts "A Is for Apple" on the newsmaga-
            zine *60 Minutes*. The broadcast publicizes the Natural
            Resources Defense Council report, "Intolerable Risk:
            Pesticides in Our Children's Food." The report and
            news story focus on the dangers, particularly to chil-
            dren, of the pesticide Alar, a growth regulator used on
            apples. Uniroyal, the maker of Alar, voluntarily with-
            draws the pesticide from the U.S. market, and the EPA
            bans the pesticide.

            Over seven thousand cows are confirmed with BSE in
            Britain.

            Two grapes in a shipment from Chile are discovered
            with cyanide. The cyanide was injected into the
            grapes at a dose too small to cause any harm, even to
            a small child. The FDA imposes a ban on Chilean fruit
            that lasts for five days.

1990   Sanitary Food Transportation Act is enacted to pro-
            hibit the practice of alternating shipments of food in
            trucks or railcars that had earlier been used to trans-
            port potentially hazardous materials.

            Nutrition Labeling and Education Act mandates the
            nutrition facts label including standardized serving
            sizes, servings per container, calories from fat, and
            amounts of other food nutrients.

            Organic Production Act defines what is meant by the
            term "organic" and sets standards for what can be
            labeled organic in the United States.

Over 14,000 cows confirmed with BSE in Britain. Twenty-six countries ban the import of British cattle and beef.

1991   Over 25,000 new cases of BSE confirmed in British cows.

1992   The first industrial irradiation facility designed exclusively for food processing opens in Tampa, Florida, and the FDA approves irradiation for poultry.

BSE is successfully transmitted by injection to animals from seven mammalian species including pigs and monkeys. Over 35,000 new cases of BSE are confirmed in Britain.

1993   In a widespread outbreak of *Escherichia coli* O157:H7 bacteria, the source is traced to tainted beef served primarily at Jack in the Box restaurants. There are 732 people who become ill, 195 are hospitalized, and 4 children die.

FDA approves recombinant bovine growth hormone (rBGH) marketed under the name Posilac. The drug, made by Monsanto, boosts milk production 5 to 20 percent.

Two British farmers, whose herds were infected with BSE, die of Creutzfeldt-Jakob disease (CJD).

National Academy of Sciences releases the report, "Pesticides in the Diets of Infants and Children." The academy concludes that fetuses, infants, and children are more susceptible than adults to toxic pesticides because their internal organs are still developing and their enzymatic, metabolic, and immune systems may provide less natural protection than those of adults.

1994   Vermont becomes the first state in the nation to mandate labeling for dairy products from cows injected

1994
(cont.)   with rBGH. The International Dairy Foods Association sues Vermont, stating that "the mandatory labeling of milk products derived from supplemented
cows will have the inherent effect of causing consumers to believe that such products are different
from and inferior to milk products from unsupple-
mented cows" (Lyman 115). Although Vermont wins
in District Court, the Circuit Court suspends the state
law on appeal.

1995   The HACCP approach to seafood inspection is adopted
by the FDA.

Ninth Circuit of the U.S. Court of Appeals dismisses a
lawsuit against CBS by apple growers claiming that
the 1989 *60 Minutes* broadcast warning of potential
health hazards of Alar was false.

1996   A group of cattlemen from Texas sues Oprah Winfrey
and Howard Lyman for food disparagement. The cattlemen claim that the two disparaged beef on the
Oprah Winfrey Show.

After ten people under the age of forty-two die of
Creutzfeldt-Jakob disease, a disease that generally
strikes much older adults, the British Secretary of
State for Health, Stephen Dornell, tells the House of
Commons that the most likely cause of these cases is
exposure to BSE from eating beef.

The FDA approves Olestra (Olean), Procter and
Gamble's controversial, indigestible fat for use in salty
foods. Olestra has been proven to cause diarrhea,
cramps, and other adverse affects.

New USDA regulations require microbial testing for
beef and poultry products. The regulations reduce the
allowable levels of various bacteria.

Animal Medicinal Drug Use Clarification Act gives
veterinarians the authority to prescribe medication

intended for use in other species. Although the American Veterinary Medical Association supports the bill, Food Animals Concerns Trust opposes it, citing concerns that untested drugs used in food animals could harm humans in the form of drug residues. Regulations require well-established veterinarian-client-patient relationships, documentation, and accountability when medications are prescribed under this act.

Food Quality Protection Act repeals the Delaney Clause, which stated that any substance that increased cancer in any dosage must not be sold. The new law permits chemical residues provided that they do not cause more than one additional cancer case for each 1 million people, and all exposures to pesticides must be shown to be safe for infants and children.

1997 Sixteen people become ill from hamburgers made from hamburger patties containing *E. coli* O157:H7, resulting in a recall of 25 million pounds of hamburger.

Food Safety—From Farm to Table: A National Food Safety Initiative, A Report to the President is released. It calls for an interagency response to food safety issues, declares foodborne illness a significant public health problem, and calls for a new early warning surveillance system.

As part of the initiative above, the Active Foodborne Disease Surveillance System, or FoodNet, is established. An interagency network of the CDC, USDA, FDA, and states participating in the CDC's Emerging Infections program, the network conducts population-based active surveillance of seven bacterial foodborne pathogens (shigella, salmonella, campylobacter, *E. coli* O157:H7, listeria, yersinia, and vibrio). Using surveys of laboratories, physicians, and the population, the network aims to determine the magnitude of diarrheal illnesses and the proportion attributable to food.

1997
(cont.)

Another network, the National Molecular Surveillance Network (PulseNet), is established by CDC in collaboration with state health departments. Taking advantage of technology that allows subtyping of *E. coli* O157:H7, routes of pathogen transmission can be traced and detected up to five times faster than by earlier epidemiological surveillance methods.

Stanley Prusiner, the developer of the prion theory, receives the Nobel Prize in Medicine or Physiology. According to Prusiner, prions are protein strands that can distort other protein strands, causing certain types of neurological diseases. They are a completely different type of infectious agent from bacteria, fungi, viruses, and parasites. Prusiner believes prions are the transmission agents for Creutzfeldt-Jakob disease, kuru, scrapie in sheep, bovine spongiform encephalopathy, and perhaps Alzheimer's disease.

The FDA ban on ruminant-to-ruminant feeding goes into effect. Cattle can no longer be fed rendered sheep or goats. However, cattle can still eat rendered horse, dog, cat, pig, chicken, turkey, or blood or fecal material from cows or chickens.

The FDA approves irradiation of beef and more intensive use of irradiation for pork and poultry.

The Canadian government consolidates all federally mandated food inspection and quarantine services into a single food inspection agency, the Canadian Food Inspection Agency (CFIA). The goal is to harmonize standards among federal, provincial, and municipal governments and make the process more efficient.

The USDA completes implementation of HACCP for meat and poultry.

Ben and Jerry's, the ice cream manufacturer, Stonyfield Farm, Whole Foods Market, and Organic

Valley Foods reach a settlement with the State of Illinois allowing food producers to state on their labels that their dairy products are rBGH free.

1998   The jury finds in favor of Howard Lyman and Oprah Winfrey in the suit filed against them by a group of Texas cattlemen claiming that they disparaged beef on the *Oprah Winfrey Show* in 1996.

1999   Twenty-one people die, five women miscarry, and seventy others are sickened when a Sara Lee–owned meat plant becomes contaminated with listeria. Fifteen million pounds of hot dogs and cold cuts are recalled.

The National Academy of Sciences warns that use of antibiotics in food animals, particularly for subthera-peutic use, increases antibiotic-resistant bacteria, making it more difficult to treat disease in humans. The academy calculates that eliminating the use of these drugs would cost consumers about $10 each per year.

2000   Irradiated beef becomes available.

Foods that have been genetically modified, grown with sewage sludge, or treated with irradiation can no longer be labeled organic.

3

Biographical Sketches

Many people from many occupations have helped to improve food safety. The following list of individuals is meant to be representative of the kinds of people active in food safety today and in the past. Among this group are activists, food safety professionals, scientists, epidemiologists, farmers, and writers.

Rachel Carson (1907–1964)

Rachel Carson grew up on a 65-acre parcel of land fifteen miles north of Pittsburgh, Pennsylvania. Her father, an aspiring real estate developer, bought the parcel with the intention of subdividing it, but Pittsburgh grew in another direction, which kept the land mostly undeveloped. Carson spent her childhood roaming the countryside and writing stories. At the age of ten she won a prize for a story from *St. Nicholas Magazine*.

In college, she majored in English until her junior year when her love of nature won out, and she switched to zoology. After college, she went to work for the Bureau of Fisheries (now part of the Department of Fish and Game) writing radio scripts about fishery and marine life.

In 1936 Carson took the civil service exam for junior aquatic biologist. She scored higher than everyone else who applied and became the first female biologist ever hired by the Bureau of Fisheries. She had many duties, but continued to write, eventually becoming the editor-in-chief of the Information Division. On the advice of her boss, she submitted one of the pieces she had written for the bureau to *Atlantic Monthly*. The magazine accepted the story, and she began to write for publication. Her first book, *Under the Sea-Wind*, was published in 1941.

In 1945, DDT became available for civilian use. It had been used during World War II in the Pacific Islands to kill malaria-causing insects and as a delousing powder in Europe. Considered a wondrous substance by many, the inventor of DDT was awarded the Nobel Prize. As part of the commercialization process, many DDT tests were conducted. Carson had observed a series of tests near her home in Maryland and approached *Reader's Digest* to propose an article about the tests. The magazine did not think the subject merited an article and Carson returned to her other writing.

The Sea Around Us was published in 1951. It described the origins and geologic aspects of the sea. It won the John Burroughs Medal, the National Book Award, and stayed on the *New York Times* bestseller list for eighty-one weeks.

In 1958, Carson received a letter from a friend, Roger Owens Huckins. Huckins owned a private bird sanctuary in Duxbury, Massachusetts. One day he found dead and dying birds a few days after a massive, unannounced spraying of DDT. Carson began researching DDT, spending four years consulting with biologists and chemists, and reviewing massive amounts of data and documentation. She wrote *Silent Spring*, carefully describing how DDT entered the food chain and accumulated in the fatty tissues of animals, including humans, causing cancer and genetic damage. She concluded that DDT and other pesticides had irrevocably harmed birds and animals and had contaminated the entire world's food supply.

Silent Spring was first serialized in the *New Yorker* in 1962. Readers all over the United States became alarmed, and the chemical industry responded sharply. Ironically, this only drew more attention to Carson's work. Carson had meticulously documented her findings; she included fifty-five pages of notes and a list of experts who had read and approved the manuscript. President John F. Kennedy instructed the President's Science Advisory Committee to examine the issues raised in the book. Their report supported the conclusions of the book and vindicated Carson.

Silent Spring became a bestseller. DDT received close scrutiny from the U.S. government and was eventually banned. Carson died of breast cancer in 1964.

Ronnie Cummins (1946–)

Ronnie Cummins has been an activist since 1967 in a variety of movements, including human rights, antiwar, antinuclear, labor, and consumer issues. In the early 1990s Cummins turned his attention to food safety, sustainable agriculture, organic food standards, and genetically modified foods. He has been the director of the Beyond Beef Campaign, the Pure Food Campaign, and the Global Days of Action Against Genetic Engineering.

Today Cummins is the national director of the Organic Consumers Association, a nonprofit, public-interest organization working to build a healthy, safe, and sustainable system of food production and consumption in the United States and the world. Cummins believes consumers' struggle for safe food is about more than staying healthy; it is also about whether people in the United States control the democratic process or whether corporations do. Perhaps because of this belief, he is most effective as a grassroots organizer. In 1998, Cummins organized the Save Organic Standards Campaign to pressure the U.S. Department of Agriculture (USDA) to strengthen the regulatory definition of what is meant by the term "organic." The USDA received more comments on this issue than on any other in recent history. As a result of the campaign, the USDA announced in 2000 that foods could not be labeled organic if they had been genetically modified.

A frequent writer, Cummins has written many articles for the alternative press, five children's books on Cuba and Central America, and a book on genetically modified food designed to help consumers avoid genetically engineered products at the grocery store.

Nancy Donley (1954–)

Nancy Donley lost her son, Alex, to hemolytic uremic syndrome (HUS) that he contracted from eating a hamburger tainted with *E. coli* O157:H7. Alex was six years old and died quickly, just four days after eating the meat. Donley, who had never been involved in any political organization before, heard about Safe Tables Our Priority (STOP) from a pediatrician who had treated her son.

She quickly joined and began lobbying for STOP. Today Donley spends twenty to twenty-five hours a week working for STOP as the unpaid president in addition to her job as a real estate broker. With the determination that netted her a degree in marketing after eleven years of night school, Donley, along with Mary Heersink and others at STOP, has pursued legislation and policy changes that have improved the safety of the U.S. food supply. STOP is largely credited with obtaining the policy change requiring HACCP and microbial testing of meats in 1996.

Donley is currently working with STOP on controlling pathogens at the farm and animal level so that pathogens don't contaminate manure used on crops, improving the foods children eat in school lunch programs where contracts usually go to the lowest bidder, and improving producer attitudes toward food safety. As a lobbyist, she is discouraged that many producers treat safety regulations as a "horse trade" instead of as an integral part of their business ethic. Some producers want to adopt certain safety regulations in exchange for removing other safety regulations. There is also a pervasive "blame the consumer" attitude. Instead of presenting consumers with untainted food, some producers blame consumers if they don't cook food adequately to kill bacteria. Donley hopes that one day there will be no need for STOP and it can cease operations.

Patricia Griffin

Patricia Griffin graduated from the University of Pennsylvania School of Medicine and stayed for internship and residency in gastroenterology. After completing a variety of research fellowships in gastroenterology, Griffin went to work for the Centers for Disease Control in the Epidemic Intelligence Service (EIS).

As an officer in the EIS, Griffin did extensive fieldwork throughout the United States as well as Thailand, Kenya, Lesotho, Brazil, Guatemala, Zambia, and Japan. In the 1980s, she became intrigued by *E. coli* O157:H7 and began conducting research. In 1983 another scientist, Mohamed Karmali, proposed that hemolytic uremic syndrome (HUS) was linked to exposure to *E. coli* O157:H7. The syndrome was first recognized in 1955, and many possible causes had been proposed. Griffin began calling pediatric nephrologists to ask them to look for the pathogen in their patients' stools. Although doctors weren't very receptive to looking for *E. coli* O157:H7, Griffin persisted and further believed that the pathogen was an important cause of bloody diarrhea.

In 1987, Marguerite Neill and Phillip Tarr did a study in Seattle showing that most cases of HUS were related to *E. coli*

O157:H7. Griffin then directed the CDC's efforts to control the disease, informing physicians of the connection to *E. coli* O157:H7, working with labs to test for the pathogen, and following up on cases around the country. In 1993, when the western states epidemic occurred, Griffin had the knowledge of the disease and the skills of an epidemiologist to identify the probable cause of the outbreak. After the outbreak, Griffin and the members of Safe Tables Our Priority (STOP) campaigned successfully to make infection with *E. coli* O157:H7 a disease that must be reported to health departments. Griffin is now director of the Foodborne and Diarrheal Diseases Branch of the CDC.

Mary Heersink

Mary Heersink led a typical suburban life as the mother of four children until 1992 when one of her sons ate undercooked hamburger at a Boy Scouts outing and developed hemolytic uremic syndrome (HUS). HUS is a complication that can develop from poisoning by *E. coli* O157:H7. Marnix Heersink, Heersink's husband and an ophthalmologist, probably saved his son's life by researching HUS and connecting his son's doctors to a hematologist familiar with the disease. Although Damion Heersink's case was severe, he made an impressive recovery.

During the five weeks Damion spent in the hospital, Heersink began to research the cause of the illness. Heersink read widely about the syndrome and its causes and became infuriated that USDA standards and procedures were not sufficient to prevent tainted meat from entering the food supply. She began to network with other parents of children who suffered from HUS, faxing medical articles to the parents of sick children, and formed Safe Tables Our Priority (STOP) with other victims of foodborne illness.

She worked tirelessly for STOP, appearing before commissions, traveling overseas to investigate other countries' practices, meeting with USDA officials, testifying before Congress, and giving interviews to the news media. Largely through the efforts of Heersink and the other parents of STOP, the USDA changed meat handling laws in 1996 to incorporate Hazard Analysis and Critical Control Points (HACCP), which requires microbial testing and performance standards for fresh and processed meats and poultry.

Fred Kirschenmann (1935–)

Fred Kirschenmann grew up on the North Dakota farm his father started in 1930. Kirschenmann left the farm and became a professor of religious history. While teaching in 1970, he was very impressed with a student's essay about how farming with heavy nitrogen fertilizers was causing deterioration of the soil. Six years later in 1976, Kirschenmann's father, Ted, suffered a heart attack. Fred offered to come home and run the farm provided he could convert it to organic agriculture.

All of Kirschenmann's neighbors thought organic farming wouldn't work, but he persisted. Using a variety of techniques including crop rotation, composting cattle manure to use as fertilizer, planting legumes to build the soil, and not planting sunflowers in the blackbirds' flight path, Kirschenmann was able to make the farm a commercial success. At 3,100 acres, his is the largest organic farm in the country. It is also a very productive farm with per acre yields the same or better than surrounding conventionally farmed fields.

Kirschenmann's success combining large-scale farming with sustainable, organic practices that are economically viable has given a huge boost to organic farming, even interesting the USDA in his methods. Conventional farmers are beginning to adopt some of the methods of sustainable agriculture, reducing their dependency on pesticides that cause pollution, are dangerous to farmworkers, and are potentially harmful to consumers. Besides running the farm, Kirschenmann is very active in the sustainable agriculture movement, traveling around the country during the winter promoting sustainable methods.

Alice Lakey (1857–1935)

Alice Lakey was born in Shanesville, Ohio. Her father was a Methodist minister and an insurance broker. Alice's mother died when Lakey was six years old. She attended public school until the age of fourteen when her father hired a private tutor for her. Lakey had a talent for singing and moved to Europe, performing on many occasions in the United Kingdom. After nearly ten years of living abroad, she returned to the United States for health reasons. A few years after her return, she and her father moved to Cranford, New Jersey. She was active in many civic causes in

Cranford, including successfully encouraging the city fathers to establish a school, fire department, and baby clinic.

When her father became ill, Lakey was unable to find unadulterated foods for him and herself. She joined the Domestic Science Unit of the Village Improvement Association and became president shortly thereafter. In 1903 Lakey wrote to Secretary of Agriculture James Wilson to get literature and a recommendation of someone who could speak to the club. He suggested Harvey Wiley (see below), then a chemist for the Department of Agriculture and the most active government worker interested in food purity issues. Wiley was quite actively trying to improve food standards. The connection with Wiley may have been what inspired Lakey to work on her goals at the national level; in 1904 she persuaded the Cranford Village Improvement Association and the New Jersey Federation of Women's Clubs to petition Congress to enact the Pure Food Bill.

In an effort to broaden support for the bill, Lakey approached the National Consumers League to support the pure food cause. The league decided to investigate the conditions under which food was prepared and the working conditions of food workers. Lakey was appointed to head the investigation committee in 1905.

The committee became known as the Pure Food Committee. The group created an activist network of the nation's pure food, drink, and drug advocates, forming a coalition of members from many organizations. Using the information from the Pure Food Committee, the league was able to articulate definite consumer objectives and speak with authority for U.S. consumers.

Lakey and Wiley met with President Roosevelt in 1905 to urge his support for the Pure Food Bill. Roosevelt told the pair that he would support the bill if they obtained signed letters to Congress. Lakey and others influenced over one million women to write letters supporting the bill.

After the bill passed in 1906, Lakey continued to work for pure food issues, pressuring Congress to fund the agency to enforce the bill and to pass the Pure Milk Bill. She continued this work until 1919 when her father died, and she took his place as manager of the trade journal he had founded, *Insurance*.

Lakey was the first woman to be listed in *Who's Who* and was named to the National Academy of Social Sciences for her work. She died of heart failure in 1935.

Antonie van Leeuwenhoek (1623–1723)

Leeuwenhoek was a Dutch tradesman with no higher education. Nevertheless, he became interested in microscopes and began making his own. The microscopes of the day were compound (made of more than one lens, similar to microscopes of today) but their magnification was only twenty to thirty times. Leeuwenhoek ground his own lenses and made microscopes by mounting the lens in a hole in a brass plate. The specimen was mounted on a sharp stick that was mounted up in front of the lens. The position and focus were adjusted with two screws. As the microscope was very small, approximately three to four inches, it had to be held close to the eye and it was difficult to use.

However, using his well-made lenses and special lighting techniques that he never revealed, Leeuwenhoek was able to magnify objects over two hundred times. He took great interest in looking at objects with his microscope and discovered bacteria, free-living and parasitic microscopic protists, sperm cells, blood cells, microscopic nematodes, and rotifers, as well as many other organisms.

The prevailing theory of the time was that low forms of animal life could appear spontaneously. Leeuwenhoek studied the weevils of granaries and was able to show that weevils are grubs hatched from eggs deposited by winged insects and not bred from wheat. At one point he examined the plaque from his teeth and was disturbed at the abundant life living in his mouth. In 1673, Leeuwenhoek started writing to the Royal Society of London describing his discoveries. Not much of an artist, he hired an illustrator to draw the microbes he saw. Although he had no formal scientific training, the Royal Society was so pleased with his discoveries that they made him a full-fledged member.

Leeuwenhoek continued working up until shortly before his death in 1723. He is considered the father of microbiology.

Howard Lyman (1938–)

Lyman was born in Montana and grew up on his family's organic dairy farm with his brother, Dick. He attended Montana State University, studying agriculture, including the business aspects of running a farm and the use of chemical fertilizers to boost productivity. After college, Lyman joined the army. Lyman liked the army, but his only brother, Dick, was dying of Hodgkin's disease, and their father was getting too old to run the farm by himself, so Lyman returned home to run the farm.

After studying the farm's books, Lyman decided the organic dairy operation was not profitable enough. He decided to use deficit financing to expand the acreage of the farm and to convert to chemical-based farming techniques.

He gradually increased his grain yield and started a feedlot operation, buying cattle and raising them for slaughter. Although he increased his acreage forty-fold, and increased his crop yields dramatically, it was almost impossible to make the farm profitable; the chemicals were expensive to use, and each year he had to use more chemicals and antibiotics to achieve the same result. The $5 million–a–year operation was taking a profound toll on the farm. The soil, once rich, loamy, and worm-filled, was crumbly and thin as sand. The worms were gone and the trees were dying.

In 1979 Lyman was diagnosed with a tumor on his spinal column. Facing probable paralysis, Lyman committed himself to restoring his family's farm to the way it was. During his long recuperation he planned a strategy. He began using integrated pest management techniques (IPM). IPM is a combination of organic farming methods and chemical techniques. Sprays are used in combination with nonchemical techniques, such as using beneficial insects like ladybugs to eat unwanted pests.

Lyman ran for Congress in 1982. Toward the end of the campaign, the bank foreclosed on his farm. Lyman lost the election by a small margin and was forced to sell off most of his holdings.

In 1983 he began working for the Montana Farmer's Union and went to Washington, D.C., as a lobbyist for them in 1987. While there, he successfully lobbied for the National Organic Standards Act and then for the funds to finance the act's administration.

In 1990, Lyman became a vegetarian for environmental, humanitarian, and health reasons. He served as president of the International Vegetarian Union and was invited to appear on the *Oprah Winfrey Show* in 1996. While on the show, Lyman discussed ruminant-to-ruminant feeding (the practice of sending leftovers from the slaughter process to rendering plants and feeding the rendered animal protein to cattle) and its link to mad cow disease. Lyman and Winfrey were sued for food disparagement by a group of Texas cattle ranchers. The jury decided in favor of Lyman and Winfrey in 1998.

Since the suit, Lyman founded Voice for a Viable Future, a campaign to educate people about sustainable agriculture and the dangers of current methods of food production.

Helen McNab Miller (1862–1949)

Helen Miller was born in Zanesville, Ohio, and studied at Stanford University, the University of Nevada, and the University of Missouri. A home economist at the Agricultural College in Columbia, Missouri, Miller had a strong professional interest in food purity issues.

As a member of the General Federation of Women's Clubs (GFWC), she was known as an energetic club woman and became chair of the pure food subcommittee. As part of her work as a home economist, she worked with many government officials and committees on pure food, drink, and milk issues. This government experience was rare among women at the time and gave Miller a unique ability to help the club set and accomplish politically viable goals. Miller advocated firm but fair legislation. She was described as tall, stately, and an accomplished speaker with a carefully modulated voice.

When President Roosevelt told Alice Lakey and Harvey Wiley to produce letters to Congress in support of the pure food legislation, Miller was assigned the task of soliciting letters from the midwestern United States. At the GFWC biennial convention in St. Paul in June 1906, Miller requested that each delegation send telegrams to their representatives in the House and Senate, the Speaker of the House, and to President Roosevelt urging swift passage of the Pure Food Bill. After Miller read a summary of the terrible state of food, drugs, and alcohol in the United States, the telegrams poured into Washington.

After the bill passed, Wiley named Lakey and Miller as outstanding leaders of the crusade. Miller continued to work on food purity issues, securing the passage of a pure milk bill in Missouri in 1907. She later moved to Kalispell, Montana. Little is known about the remainder of her life.

Michael Osterholm (1953–)

After graduating from medical school, Osterholm went to work for the Minnesota Department of Health. He worked in various positions until he became state epidemiologist in 1985. In his position as chief, Osterholm improved the level of surveillance in Minnesota, creating a reporting system more advanced than most other states. He led many investigations of outbreaks of foodborne disease and did extensive research in epidemiology. His team was the first to call attention to the changing epidemiology of foodborne illness.

As the chair of the Emerging Infections Committee of the Infectious Disease Society of America, Osterholm has become an expert not only in foodborne illness but also biological terrorism and antimicrobial resistance. Osterholm has been a principal investigator for the Centers for Disease Control (CDC) and a consultant for the National Institutes of Health, the FDA, and the World Health Organization.

In 1999, Osterholm left the state of Minnesota to found ICAN, Inc., an Internet-based resource for health professionals. Designed to aid in diagnosis and prescription of drugs, the database can be used to help doctors and others treat infectious diseases.

Louis Pasteur (1822–1895)

Louis Pasteur, the son of a tanner, spent a carefree childhood in France. It was not until later that he developed an interest in science, earning a bachelor's degree in science in 1842, followed by master's and doctorate degrees in 1845 and 1847 respectively.

In 1854 Pasteur became dean of the new science faculty at the University of Lillie. As dean, he introduced programs to create a bridge between science and industry, including taking his students to factories, supervising practical courses, and starting evening classes for young workmen. Perhaps because of the connections he made to industry, a businessman inquired about producing alcohol from grain and beet sugar. This began his study of fermentation.

In 1857 he announced that fermentation was the result of the activity of minute organisms. If fermentation failed, it was because the necessary organism was missing or unable to grow properly. As he continued his research, he proved that food decomposes when placed in contact with germs present in the air. He discovered that spoilage could be prevented if the microbes already present in foodstuffs were destroyed and the sterilized material was protected against later contamination.

A practical man, Pasteur applied his theory to food and drinks, developing a heat treatment called pasteurization. He was able to aid the French wine industry, which was trying to solve the problem of wine going sour when it was transported, and his process eliminated the serious health threats of bovine tuberculosis, brucellosis, and other milk-borne diseases.

Pasteur's interest in bacteria also led him to study diseases. After he had determined the natural history of anthrax, a fatal disease of cattle, he concluded that anthrax was caused by a particular bacillus. He suggested giving anthrax in a mild form to animals to inoculate them against a more severe reaction. He tested his hypothesis on sheep, inoculating twenty-five with a mild case of anthrax. A few days later he inoculated the same twenty-five plus twenty-five untreated sheep with a virulent strain of the bacteria. He left ten sheep completely untreated. As Pasteur believed would happen, the twenty-five sheep who had been vaccinated survived, but the twenty-five who were given the virulent bacteria died. Pasteur continued to study diseases and was able to develop vaccines for chicken cholera, smallpox, and rabies before his death in 1895.

Stanley Prusiner (1942–)

Prusiner was born in Des Moines, Iowa, and went to the University of Pennsylvania where he earned a bachelor's degree in 1964 and a medical degree in 1968. He started a residency at the University of California–San Francisco in neurology, intending to enter private practice after graduation. One of his patients died of Creutzfeldt-Jakob disease (CJD) and Prusiner decided to stay at UCSF to research the disease instead of entering private practice.

Over the course of his research, Prusiner determined that an abnormal protein, which Prusiner dubbed a prion (for protinaceous infectious particle), caused the infection. The prion was a previously unrecognized infectious agent, different from bacteria, viruses, and parasites. A prion is a protein that has the same amino acids as a normal protein but is shaped differently. It is the different shape that Prusiner believes causes certain brain disorders, including other spongiform encephalopathies like kuru, a disease of human cannibals, scrapie in sheep, and bovine spongiform encephalopathy (BSE). In 1984, Prusiner and his group identified fifteen amino acids at the end of the prion protein. This discovery was enough for other labs to identify the gene for producing the prion protein in both healthy and infected mice and hamsters.

In 1992, Prusiner, with Charles Weissmann of the University of Zurich, was able to show that lab mice stripped of the prion gene became immune to prion-linked diseases. Although some scientists don't believe that the deformed prion is the infectious agent, in 1997 Prusiner was awarded the Nobel Prize for Medicine or Physiology. He continues to study prion diseases, and this research will hopefully bring us closer to a cure.

John Robbins (1947–)

John Robbins, the only son of one of the founders of the Baskin-Robbins ice cream empire, was groomed from childhood to take over the family business. Early in his college career at the University of California–Berkeley, Robbins decided that he didn't want to work for the family business, in part because he felt high-fat ice creams contributed to the ill health of Americans. He walked away from the extensive wealth and position his family offered to pursue his own ideas. After a stint as a psychotherapist, Robbins became interested in the way animals were raised for food, the health consequences of the typical American diet, and the environmental consequences of eating animal products. Robbins wrote *Diet for a New America* in 1987 to explain his beliefs. In the book, Robbins explains how food choices affect human health, showing that vegetarians suffer from heart disease and other degenerative diseases at lower rates than meat eaters. The book was an international bestseller and was nominated for a Pulitzer Prize.

He founded Earth-Save Foundation, an organization devoted to helping protect the environment through encouraging others to adopt a plant-based diet. For one of his foundation's projects he goes to schools to talk about vegetarian nutrition. Many of the materials schools use to teach nutrition come from the National Dairy Council and promote animal-based diets. Earth-Save has also worked with school districts to offer meatless and no-animal-product choices on school lunch menus.

Ironically, Robbins's father has now adopted many of the dietary principles his son, John, espouses at the recommendation of his doctor. Robbins is a frequent speaker, giving about a hundred talks a year all over the world.

Upton Sinclair (1878–1968)

Upton Sinclair was born in Baltimore, Maryland. Although both his parents came from middle- and upper-middle-class backgrounds, his father was an unsuccessful salesman. His lack of success propelled the family into poverty. Sinclair lived in bug-ridden boardinghouses with his parents and later alternated between this environment and Baltimore society with his mother's well-off relatives. Sinclair's father turned more and more to alcohol, and Sinclair was often sent to bars to retrieve his father. The contrast between his luxury with his relatives and the poverty he saw with his parents led to a great social awareness and a desire to increase social justice. After completing college at eighteen, he became a hack writer of young men's adventure stories. He was interested in social issues, however, and his early serious novels began to show evidence of his conversion to socialism.

In 1904 Sinclair was commissioned by a widely circulating socialist weekly, *Appeal to Reason*, to investigate labor conditions in the Chicago stockyards. With a $500 stipend, he spent seven weeks in Chicago and returned to Princeton, New Jersey, to write *The Jungle*. The novel documented alarmingly unsanitary conditions in the Chicago stockyards and the hard life of the immigrants who worked there. In 1905 it was serialized in *Appeal to Reason*. Although enormously popular in serial form, Sinclair had a difficult time getting the novel published in book form. It was rejected by several book publishers, and Sinclair prepared to publish it himself. Doubleday finally agreed to publish it if the conditions Sinclair wrote about could be adequately documented. They sent a lawyer to Chicago who was able to substantiate Sinclair's findings.

In 1906 *The Jungle* was published. Within two months it was selling in Britain and had been translated into seventeen languages. People were outraged at the lax standards for processing meat. The publicity that Sinclair created was enough to get the Pure Food and Drug Bill and the Beef Inspection Bill passed. This legislation had originally been proposed in 1902, but it took public sentiment and pressure from President Roosevelt to get the bill passed in 1906.

Sinclair ran for governor in California in 1934 with the slogan "End Poverty in California." He was narrowly defeated and retired from politics. Although in later life Sinclair continued to write about many social issues, he is best known for *The Jungle*, and he had more impact on food safety than any other issue.

David Theno (1950–)

David Theno grew up in rural northern Illinois raising farm animals. Although he was planning to be a veterinarian, he found himself enjoying the blend of science and business in the Animal Sciences and Foods Group at the University of Illinois. When he was invited to stay for a doctorate degree with the group, he skipped veterinary school and earned a Ph.D. in muscle biology in 1977. As a food technologist implementing new technologies, Theno earned a reputation as an effective troubleshooter. Within a few years he was working at Armor Foods as the director of Product Quality and Technology where he applied a troubleshooter's eye to continually making processing safer.

At Foster Farms in the 1980s, Theno developed and implemented the first comprehensive HACCP system in the poultry industry and was able to decrease salmonella counts to less than one-third the counts at other plants.

Theno started a consulting business designing and implementing HACCP systems for companies all over the country. When tainted hamburger served at Jack in the Box restaurants in 1993 sickened hundreds and killed four toddlers, Theno was asked to take over food safety operations. By 1994, Jack in the Box, under Theno's direction, had implemented HACCP standards that exceeded the Model Food Code of the Food and Drug Administration. Today, Jack in the Box leads the fast food industry in food safety. Theno has achieved this through both his technical knowledge and his ability to design systems where workers, often low skilled, feel a sense of personal responsibility for serving a safe product. Theno credits the high level of integrity in the corporate cultures of the companies he's worked at. These companies commit to "doing it right, not just doing a good enough job," said Theno.

Theno's HACCP system at Jack in the Box continues to evolve; and every six months, new procedures are designed with input from the restaurant managers. But Theno hasn't just improved food safety at his own company. The company invites others in the industry to visit and learn Jack in the Box's HACCP system. He has also served on the USDA's Meat and Poultry Committee and the National Committee for Microbial Standards. Theno and Jack in the Box's commitment to food safety serve as role models for proactive food safety management at the corporate level.

Harvey Wiley (1844–1930)

Harvey Wiley was born in a log cabin on a frontier Indiana farm. Wiley's father, Preston Wiley, was a teacher at a subscription school and took his son to school with him when Harvey turned four. Preston drew a chalk square in the classroom for his son. Harvey was instructed to stay in the square and learned to read through his father's instruction. He attended Hanover College and served in the army during the U.S. Civil War. He wanted to become a doctor to help people, and he believed that an essential part of living a healthy life was eating healthful food. In medical school, he became interested in preventative medicine, and he believed that moderate eating was important for health.

Wiley demonstrated a talent for analytical chemistry in college and medical school and never practiced medicine. He earned a doctorate degree in chemistry from Harvard University, and became a researcher and professor at Northwestern Christian College and Purdue University. At Northwestern Christian, Wiley taught chemistry with student labs, something novel at that time. At Purdue University, Wiley became the state chemist for Indiana, and studied the syrup and sugar produced by the hydrolysis of cornstarch. This corn sugar was frequently used as a cheap adulterant for cane and maple syrup products. At that time there were no regulations requiring accurate labeling of contents. Wiley lobbied the Indiana state legislature to require manufacturers to label contents.

In 1883, Wiley was offered an appointment with the United States Department of Agriculture as a chemist. He was hired to help establish a U.S. sugar industry, but he continued to be interested in food purity issues. Mainly through his work, pure food bills were introduced to Congress throughout the 1880s and 1890s but none passed. He was one of the leading chemists of the day and helped found the Association of Official Analytical Chemists in 1891, which still offers an award in his name.

In 1902, Wiley organized a volunteer team of healthy young men called the "poison squad" who volunteered to eat all their meals in Wiley's special kitchen. Wiley gave the men large doses of the preservatives and adulterants in common use at the time to determine what ill effects they might cause. Testing one substance at a time, Wiley was able to demonstrate the unhealthful effects of many substances.

The "poison squad" garnered considerable publicity. Upton Sinclair's book, *The Jungle,* came out in 1906, exposing the unsanitary conditions in the nation's meatpacking plants. The steady pressure from Wiley coupled with increasing public pressure led to the passage of the Pure Food and Drug Act of 1906. Wiley was appointed to oversee the administration of the act and stayed in government service until 1912.

Recruited by Good Housekeeping in 1912, Wiley set up the magazine's Bureau of Foods, Sanitation, and Health. He lobbied for tougher government inspection of meat, pure butter unadulterated by water, and unadulterated wheat flour, which growers were mixing with other grains. At Good Housekeeping, his bureau analyzed food products and published its findings. They gave the Good Housekeeping "Tested and Approved" seal to those products that met their standards of purity.

Before his death in 1930 at the age of 86, Wiley had authored a number of books, contributed to the passage of the maternal health bill, which allocated federal funds for improved infant care, and helped secure legislation to keep refined sugar pure and unadulterated.

Craig Wilson (1948–)

Craig Wilson was working at Frigoscandia in Redmond, Washington, in 1993 when four children died and many more got sick from eating tainted hamburger at Jack in the Box restaurants. Some of the children were friends of his own children. Frigoscandia manufactures equipment for a variety of applications including food-processing plants. Wilson understood the mechanism of the *E. coli* O157:H7 poisoning; bacteria that is often present in the gut of cows had gotten onto the carcass during processing and had tainted many pounds of hamburger when the carcass was ground up. *E. coli* O157:H7 is so virulent that as little as one bacterial organism can cause illness. If bacteria from one animal contaminates a carcass, it can affect thousands of pounds of meat, because hamburger is processed in such large batches.

Wilson decided that what was needed was a better way to treat carcasses so that even if some bacteria got onto the carcass, the bacteria could be killed before the meat was ground up. Wilson came up with the idea of steaming the carcasses in a quick burst. The process would be long enough to kill any bacteria contaminating the surface but not long enough to cook the meat.

Wilson approached one of Frigoscandia's customers, Cargill, one of the largest meat processors, and Cargill's Jerry Leising worked with Wilson. Together they approached Randy Phebus at Kansas State University and the three of them were able to turn Wilson's idea into a commercially viable process. Wilson stayed at Frigoscandia until 1998 and is now director of Food Safety at Costco. The process continues to be perfected. The team has recently adapted the approach for pork.

4

Facts and Statistics

The U.S. Food and Drug Administration, Center for Food Safety and Applied Nutrition, has created the Bad Bug Book, an online, frequently updated summary of the causes of food-borne illnesses. Each cause includes the nature of the disease, including symptoms, onset time, infective dose, relative frequency of disease, and selected disease outbreaks. When viewed online, links are provided to the Centers for Disease Control and Prevention's *Morbidity and Mortality Weekly Report* and relevant abstracts available on Medline, the National Library of Medicine's online medical database. The document can be viewed online at http://vm.cfsan.fda.gov/~mow/intro.html.

Bad Bug Book: Foodborne Pathogenic Microorganisms and Natural Toxins Handbook

Salmonella spp.

1. Name of the Organism   *Salmonella* spp. Salmonella is a rod-shaped, motile bacterium—nonmotile exceptions *S. gallinarum* and *S. pullorum*—nonspore-forming and Gram-negative. There is a widespread occurrence in animals, especially in poultry and swine. Environmental sources of the organism include water, soil, insects, factory surfaces, kitchen surfaces, animal feces, raw meats, raw poultry, and raw seafood, to name only a few.

2. Nature of Acute Disease   *S. typhi* and the paratyphoid bacteria normally cause septicemia and produce typhoid or typhoid-like fever in humans. Other forms of salmonellosis generally produce milder symptoms.

3. Nature of Disease

Acute symptoms—Nausea, vomiting, abdominal cramps, mild diarrhea, fever, and headache. Chronic consequences—arthritic symptoms may follow 3–4 weeks after onset of acute symptoms.

Onset time—6–48 hours.

Infective dose—As few as 15–20 cells; depends upon age and health of host and strain differences among the members of the genus.

Duration of symptoms—Acute symptoms may last for 1 to 2 days or may be prolonged, again depending on host factors, ingested dose, and strain characteristics.

Cause of disease—Penetration and passage of Salmonella organisms from gut lumen into epithelium of small intestine where inflammation occurs; there is evidence that an enterotoxin may be produced, perhaps within the enterocyte.

4. Diagnosis of Human Illness

Serological identification of culture isolated from stool.

5. Associated Foods

Raw meats, poultry, eggs, milk and dairy products, fish, shrimp, frog legs, yeast, coconut, sauces and salad dressing, cake mixes, cream-filled desserts and toppings, dried gelatin, peanut butter, cocoa, and chocolate.

Various Salmonella species have long been isolated from the outside of egg shells. The present situation with *S. enteritidis* is complicated by the presence of the organism inside the egg, in the yolk. This and other information strongly suggest vertical transmission, i.e., deposition of the organism in the yolk by an infected layer hen prior to shell deposition. Foods other than eggs have also caused outbreaks of *S. enteritidis* disease.

6. Relative Frequency of Disease

It is estimated that from 2 to 4 million cases of salmonellosis occur in the U.S. annually.

The incidence of salmonellosis appears to be rising both in the U.S. and in other industrialized nations. *S. enteritidis* isolations from humans have shown a dramatic rise in the past decade, particularly in the northeast United States (6-fold or more), and the increase in human infections is spreading south and west, with sporadic outbreaks in other regions.

7. Complications S. *typhi* and S. *paratyphi* A, B, and C produce typhoid and typhoid-like fever in humans. Various organs may be infected, leading to lesions. The fatality rate of typhoid fever is 10% compared to less than 1% for most forms of salmonellosis. S. *dublin* has a 15% mortality rate when septicemic in the elderly, and S. *enteritidis* is demonstrating approximately a 3.6% mortality rate in hospital/nursing home outbreaks, with the elderly being particularly affected.

Salmonella septicemia has been associated with subsequent infection of virtually every organ system.

Postenteritis reactive arthritis and Reiter's syndrome have also been reported to occur generally after 3 weeks. Reactive arthritis may occur with a frequency of about 2% of culture-proven cases. Septic arthritis, subsequent or coincident with septicemia, also occurs and can be difficult to treat.

8. Target Populations All age groups are susceptible, but symptoms are most severe in the elderly, infants, and the infirm. AIDS patients suffer salmonellosis frequently (estimated 20-fold more than general population) and suffer from recurrent episodes.

9. Foods Analysis Methods have been developed for many foods having prior history of Salmonella contamination. Although conventional culture methods require 5 days for presumptive results, several rapid methods are available which require only 2 days.

10. Selected Outbreaks In 1985, a salmonellosis outbreak involving 16,000 confirmed cases in 6 states was caused by low fat and whole milk from one Chicago dairy. This was the largest outbreak of foodborne salmonellosis in the U.S. FDA inspectors discovered that the pasteurization equipment had been modified to facilitate the running off of raw milk, resulting in the pasteurized milk being contaminated with raw milk under certain conditions. The dairy has subsequently disconnected the cross-linking line. Persons on antibiotic therapy were more apt to be affected in this outbreak.

In August and September, 1985, S. *enteritidis* was isolated from employees and patrons of three restaurants of a chain in Maryland. The outbreak in one restaurant had at least 71 illnesses resulting in 17 hospitalizations. Scrambled eggs from a breakfast bar were epidemiologically implicated in this outbreak and in possibly one other of the three restaurants. The plasmid profiles of isolates from patients at all three restaurants matched.

The Centers for Disease Control (CDC) has recorded more than 120 outbreaks of *S. enteritidis* to date, many occurring in restaurants, and some in nursing homes, hospitals and prisons.

In 1984, 186 cases of salmonellosis *(S. enteritidis)* were reported on 29 flights to the United States on a single international airline. An estimated 2,747 passengers were affected overall. No specific food item was implicated, but food ordered from the first class menu was strongly associated with disease.

S. enteritidis outbreaks continue to occur in the U.S. The CDC estimates that 75% of those outbreaks are associated with the consumption of raw or inadequately cooked Grade A whole shell eggs. The U.S. Department of Agriculture published Regulations on February 16, 1990, in the Federal Register establishing a mandatory testing program for egg-producing breeder flocks and commercial flocks implicated in causing human illnesses. This testing should lead to a reduction in cases of gastroenteritis caused by the consumption of Grade A whole shell eggs.

Salmonellosis associated with a Thanksgiving Dinner in Nevada in 1995 is reported in MMWR 45(46):1996 Nov 22.

MMWR 45(34):1996 Aug 30 reports on several outbreaks of *Salmonella enteritidis* infection associated with the consumption of raw shell eggs in the United States from 1994 to 1995.

A report of an outbreak of Salmonella Serotype Typhimurium infection associated with the consumption of raw ground beef may be found in MMWR 44(49):1995 Dec 15.

MMWR 44(42):1995 Oct 27 reports on an outbreak of Salmonellosis associated with beef jerky in New Mexico in 1995.

The report on the outbreak of Salmonella from commercially prepared ice cream is found in MMWR 43(40):1994 Oct 14.

An outbreak of *S. enteritidis* in homemade ice cream is reported in this MMWR 43(36):1994 Sep 16.

A series of *S. enteritidis* outbreaks in California are summarized in the following MMWR 42(41):1993 Oct 22.

For information on an outbreak of Salmonella Serotype Tennessee in Powdered Milk Products and Infant Formula see this MMWR 42(26):1993 Jul 09.

Summaries of Salmonella outbreaks associated with Grade A eggs are reported in MMWR 37(32):1988 Aug 19 and MMWR 39(50):1990 Dec 21.

For more information on recent outbreaks see the *Morbidity and Mortality Weekly Reports* from CDC.

11. Education

The CDC provides an informational brochure on preventing *Salmonella enteritidis* infection.

Food Safety Facts for Consumers (July 1999)

12. Other Resources

A Loci index for genome *Salmonella enteritidis* is available from GenBank.

Clostridium botulinum

1. Name of the Organism

Clostridium botulinum is an anaerobic, Gram-positive, spore-forming rod that produces a potent neurotoxin. The spores are heat-resistant and can survive in foods that are incorrectly or minimally processed. Seven types (A, B, C, D, E, F and G) of botulism are recognized, based on the antigenic specificity of the toxin produced by each strain. Types A, B, E and F cause human botulism. Types C and D cause most cases of botulism in animals. Animals most commonly affected are wild fowl and poultry, cattle, horses and some species of fish. Although type G has been isolated from soil in Argentina, no outbreaks involving it have been recognized.

Foodborne botulism (as distinct from wound botulism and infant botulism) is a severe type of food poisoning caused by the ingestion of foods containing the potent neurotoxin formed during growth of the organism. The toxin is heat labile and can be destroyed if heated at 80 degrees C for 10 minutes or longer. The incidence of the disease is low, but the disease is of considerable concern because of its high mortality rate if not treated immediately and properly. Most of the 10 to 30 outbreaks that are reported annually in the United States are associated with inadequately processed, home-canned foods, but occasionally commercially produced foods have been involved in outbreaks. Sausages, meat products, canned vegetables, and seafood products have been the most frequent vehicles for human botulism.

The organism and its spores are widely distributed in nature. They occur in both cultivated and forest soils, bottom sediments of streams, lakes, and coastal waters, and in the intestinal tracts of fish and mammals, and in the gills and viscera of crabs and other shellfish.

2. Name of the Disease

Four types of botulism are recognized: foodborne, infant, wound, and a form of botulism whose classification is as yet undetermined. Certain foods have been reported as sources of spores in cases of infant botulism and the undetermined category; wound botulism is not related to foods.

Foodborne botulism is the name of the disease (actually a foodborne intoxication) caused by the consumption of foods containing the neurotoxin produced by *C. botulinum.*

Infant botulism, first recognized in 1976, affects infants under 12 months of age. This type of botulism is caused by the ingestion of *C. botulinum* spores which colonize and produce toxin in the intestinal tract of infants (intestinal toxemia botulism). Of the various potential environmental sources such as soil, cistern water, dust and foods, honey is the one dietary reservoir of *C. botulinum* spores thus far definitively linked to infant botulism by both laboratory and epidemiologic studies. The number of confirmed infant botulism cases has increased significantly as a result of greater awareness by health officials since its recognition in 1976. It is now internationally recognized, with cases being reported in more countries.

Wound botulism is the rarest form of botulism. The illness results when *C. botulinum* by itself or with other microorganisms infects a wound and produces toxins which reach other parts of the body via the blood stream. Foods are not involved in this type of botulism.

Undetermined category of botulism involves adult cases in which a specific food or wound source cannot be identified. It has been suggested that some cases of botulism assigned to this category might result from intestinal colonization in adults, with in vivo production of toxin. Reports in the medical literature suggest the existence of a form of botulism similar to infant botulism, but occurring in adults. In these cases, the patients had surgical alterations of the gastrointestinal tract and/or antibiotic therapy. It is proposed that these procedures may have altered the normal gut flora and allowed *C. botulinum* to colonize the intestinal tract.

3. Nature of the Disease

Infective dose—a very small amount (a few nanograms) of toxin can cause illness.

Onset of symptoms in foodborne botulism is usually 18 to 36 hours after ingestion of the food containing the toxin, although cases have varied from 4 hours to 8 days. Early signs of intoxication consist of marked lassitude, weakness and vertigo, usually followed by double vision and progressive difficulty in speaking and swallowing. Difficulty in breathing, weakness of other muscles, abdominal distention, and constipation may also be common symptoms.

Clinical symptoms of infant botulism consist of constipation that occurs after a period of normal development. This is followed by poor feeding, lethargy, weakness, pooled oral secretions, and wail or altered cry. Loss of head control is striking. Recommended treatment is primarily supportive care. Antimicrobial therapy is not recommended. Infant botulism is diagnosed by demonstrating botulinal toxins and the organism in the infant's stools.

4. Diagnosis of Human Illness

Although botulism can be diagnosed by clinical symptoms alone, differentiation from other diseases may be difficult. The most direct and effective way to confirm the clinical diagnosis of botulism in the laboratory is to demonstrate the presence of toxin in the serum or feces of the patient or in the food which the patient consumed. Currently, the most sensitive and widely used method for detecting toxin is the mouse neutralization test. This test takes 48 hours. Culturing of specimens takes 5–7 days.

5. Associated Foods

The types of foods involved in botulism vary according to food preservation and eating habits in different regions. Any food that is conducive to outgrowth and toxin production, that when processed allows spore survival, and is not subsequently heated before consumption can be associated with botulism. Almost any type of food that is not very acidic (pH above 4.6) can support growth and toxin production by *C. botulinum.* Botulinal toxin has been demonstrated in a considerable variety of foods, such as canned corn, peppers, green beans, soups, beets, asparagus, mushrooms, ripe olives, spinach, tuna fish, chicken and chicken livers and liver pate, and luncheon meats, ham, sausage, stuffed eggplant, lobster, and smoked and salted fish.

6. Frequency

The incidence of the disease is low, but the mortality rate is high if not treated immediately and properly. There are generally between 10 and 30 outbreaks a year in the United States. Some cases of botulism may go undiagnosed because symptoms are transient or mild, or misdiagnosed as Guillain-Barre syndrome.

7. The Usual Course of Disease and Complications

Botulinum toxin causes flaccid paralysis by blocking motor nerve terminals at the myoneural junction. The flaccid paralysis progresses symmetrically downward, usually starting with the eyes and face, to the throat, chest and extremities. When the diaphragm and chest muscles become fully involved, respiration is inhibited and death from asphyxia results. Recommended treatment for foodborne botulism includes early administration of botulinal antitoxin (available from CDC) and intensive supportive care (including mechanical breathing assistance).

8. Target Populations

All people are believed to be susceptible to the foodborne intoxication.

9. Food Analysis

Since botulism is foodborne and results from ingestion of the toxin of *C. botulinum*, determination of the source of an outbreak is based on detection and identification of toxin in the food involved. The most widely accepted method is the injection of extracts of the food into passively immunized mice (mouse neutralization test). The test takes 48 hours. This analysis is followed by culturing all suspect food in an enrichment medium for the detection and isolation of the causative organism. This test takes 7 days.

10. Selected Outbreaks

Two separate outbreaks of botulism have occurred involving commercially canned salmon. Restaurant foods such as sauteed onions, chopped bottled garlic, potato salad made from baked potatoes and baked potatoes themselves have been responsible for a number of outbreaks. Also, smoked fish, both hot and cold-smoke (e.g., Kapchunka) have caused outbreaks of type E botulism.

In October and November, 1987, 8 cases of type E botulism occurred, 2 in New York City and 6 in Israel. All 8 patients had consumed Kapchunka, an uneviscerated, dry-salted, air-dried, whole whitefish. The product was made in New York City and some of it was transported by individuals to Israel. All 8 patients with botulism developed symptoms within 36 hours of consuming the Kapchunka. One female died, 2 required breathing assistance, 3 were treated therapeutically with antitoxin, and 3 recovered spontaneously. The Kapchunka involved in this outbreak contained high levels of type E botulinal toxin despite salt levels that exceeded those sufficient to inhibit *C. botulinum* type E outgrowth. One possible explanation was that the fish contained low salt levels when air-dried at room temperature, became toxic, and then were re-brined. Regulations were published to prohibit the processing, distribution and sale of Kapchunka and Kapchunka-type products in the United States.

A bottled chopped garlic-in-oil mix was responsible for three cases of botulism in Kingston, N.Y. Two men and a woman were hospitalized with botulism after consuming a chopped garlic-in-oil mix that had been used in a spread for garlic bread. The bottled chopped garlic relied solely on refrigeration to ensure safety and did not contain any additional antibotulinal additives or barriers. The FDA has ordered companies to stop making the product and to withdraw from the market any garlic-in-oil mix which does not include microbial inhibitors or acidifying agents and does not require refrigeration for safety.

Since botulism is a life-threatening disease, FDA always initiates a Class I recall.

An incident of foodborne botulism in Oklahoma is reported in MMWR 44(11):1995 Mar 24.

A botulism type B outbreak in Italy associated with eggplant in oil is reported in MMWR 44(2):1995 Jan 20.

The botulism outbreak associated with salted fish mentioned above is reported in greater detail in MMWR 36(49):1987 Dec 18.

For more information on recent outbreaks see the *Morbidity and Mortality Weekly Reports* from CDC.

11. Education   The December 1995 issue of "FDA Consumer" has an article titled Botulism Toxin: a Poison That Can Heal which discusses Botulism toxin with an emphasis on its medical uses.

12. Other Resources   FDA Warns Against Consuming Certain Italian Mascarpone Cream Cheese Because of Potential Serious Botulism Risk (Sept. 9, 1996)

A Loci index for genome *Clostridium botulinum* is available from GenBank.

Staphylococcus aureus

1. Name of the Organism   *Staphylococcus aureus*

S. aureus is a spherical bacterium (coccus) which on microscopic examination appears in pairs, short chains, or bunched, grape-like clusters. These organisms are Gram-positive. Some strains are capable of producing a highly heat-stable protein toxin that causes illness in humans.

2. Name of Acute Disease   Staphylococcal food poisoning (staphyloentero-toxicosis; staphyloenterotoxemia) is the name of the condition caused by the enterotoxins which some strains of *S. aureus* produce.

3. Nature of the Disease   The onset of symptoms in staphylococcal food poisoning is usually rapid and in many cases acute, depending on individual susceptibility to the toxin, the amount of contaminated food eaten, the amount of toxin in the food ingested, and the general health of the victim. The most common symptoms are nausea, vomiting, retching, abdominal cramping, and prostration. Some individuals may not always demonstrate all the symptoms associated with the illness. In more severe cases, headache, muscle cramping, and transient changes in blood pressure and pulse rate may occur. Recovery generally takes two days. However, it is not unusual for complete recovery to take three days and sometimes longer in severe cases.

Infective dose—a toxin dose of less than 1.0 microgram in contaminated food will produce symptoms of staphylococcal intoxication. This toxin level is reached when *S. aureus* populations exceed 100,000 per gram.

4. Diagnosis of Human Illness

In the diagnosis of staphylococcal foodborne illness, proper interviews with the victims and gathering and analyzing epidemiologic data are essential. Incriminated foods should be collected and examined for staphylococci. The presence of relatively large numbers of enterotoxigenic staphylococci is good circumstantial evidence that the food contains toxin. The most conclusive test is the linking of an illness with a specific food or in cases where multiple vehicles exist, the detection of the toxin in the food sample(s). In cases where the food may have been treated to kill the staphylococci, as in pasteurization or heating, direct microscopic observation of the food may be an aid in the diagnosis. A number of serological methods for determining the enterotoxigenicity of *S. aureus* isolated from foods as well as methods for the separation and detection of toxins in foods have been developed and used successfully to aid in the diagnosis of the illness. Phage typing may also be useful when viable staphylococci can be isolated from the incriminated food, from victims, and from suspected carriers such as food handlers.

5. Foods Incriminated

Foods that are frequently incriminated in staphylococcal food poisoning include meat and meat products; poultry and egg products; salads such as egg, tuna, chicken, potato, and macaroni; bakery products such as cream-filled pastries, cream pies, and chocolate eclairs; sandwich fillings; and milk and dairy products. Foods that require considerable handling during preparation and that are kept at slightly elevated temperatures after preparation are frequently involved in staphylococcal food poisoning.

Staphylococci exist in air, dust, sewage, water, milk, and food or on food equipment, environmental surfaces, humans, and animals. Humans and animals are the primary reservoirs. Staphylococci are present in the nasal passages and throats and on the hair and skin of 50 percent or more of healthy individuals. This incidence is even higher for those who associate with or who come in contact with sick individuals and hospital environments. Although food handlers are usually the main source of food contamination in food poisoning outbreaks, equipment and environmental surfaces can also be sources of contamination with *S. aureus*. Human intoxication is caused by ingesting enterotoxins produced in food by some strains of *S. aureus*, usually because the food has not been kept hot enough (60 degrees C, 140 degrees F, or above) or cold enough (7.2 degrees C, 45 degrees F, or below).

6. Frequency of Illness

The true incidence of staphylococcal food poisoning is unknown for a number of reasons, including poor responses from victims during interviews with health officials; misdiagnosis of the illness, which may be symptomatically similar to other types of food poisoning (such as vomiting caused by *Bacillus cereus* toxin); inadequate collection of samples for laboratory analyses; and improper laboratory examination. Of the bacterial pathogens causing foodborne illnesses in the U.S. (127 outbreaks, 7,082 cases recorded in 1983), 14 outbreaks involving 1,257 cases were caused by *S. aureus*. These outbreaks were followed by 11 outbreaks (1,153 cases) in 1984, 14 outbreaks (421 cases) in 1985, 7 outbreaks (250 cases) in 1986 and one reported outbreak (100 cases) in 1987.

7. Complications

Death from staphylococcal food poisoning is very rare, although such cases have occurred among the elderly, infants, and severely debilitated persons.

8. Target Population

All people are believed to be susceptible to this type of bacterial intoxication; however, intensity of symptoms may vary.

9. Analysis of Foods

For detecting trace amounts of staphylococcal enterotoxin in foods incriminated in food poisoning, the toxin must be separated from food constituents and concentrated before identification by specific precipitation with antiserum (antienterotoxin) as follows. Two principles are used for the purpose: (1) the selective adsorption of the enterotoxin from an extract of the food onto ion exchange resins and (2) the use of physical and chemical procedures for the selective removal of food constituents from the extract, leaving the enterotoxin(s) in solution. The use of these techniques and concentration of the resulting products (as much as possible) has made it possible to detect small amounts of enterotoxin in food.

There are developed rapid methods based on monoclonal antibodies (e.g., ELISA, Reverse Passive Latex Agglutination), which are being evaluated for their efficacy in the detection of enterotoxins in food. These rapid methods can detect approximately 1.0 nanogram of toxin/g of food.

10. Typical Outbreak

1,364 children became ill out of a total of 5,824 who had eaten lunch served at 16 elementary schools in Texas. The lunches were prepared in a central kitchen and transported to the schools by truck. Epidemiological studies revealed that 95% of the children who became ill had eaten a chicken salad. The afternoon of the day preceding the lunch, frozen chickens were boiled for 3 hours. After cooking, the chickens were deboned, cooled to room temperature with a fan, ground into small pieces, placed into 12-inch-deep aluminum pans and stored overnight in a walk-in refrigerator at 42–45 degrees F.

The following morning, the remaining ingredients of the salad were added and the mixture was blended with an electric mixer. The food was placed in thermal containers and transported to the various schools at 9:30 AM to 10:30 AM, where it was kept at room temperature until served between 11:30 AM and noon. Bacteriological examination of the chicken salad revealed the presence of large numbers of *S. aureus*.

Contamination of the chicken probably occurred when it was deboned. The chicken was not cooled rapidly enough because it was stored in 12-inch-deep layers. Growth of the staphylococcus probably occurred also during the period when the food was kept in the warm classrooms. Prevention of this incident would have entailed screening the individuals who deboned the chicken for carriers of the staphylococcus, more rapid cooling of the chicken, and adequate refrigeration of the salad from the time of preparation to its consumption.

11. Atypical Outbreaks

In 1989, multiple staphylococcal foodborne diseases were associated with the consumption of canned mushrooms. (CDC *Morbidity and Mortality Weekly Report*, June 23, 1989, Vol. 38, #24.)

Starkville, Mississippi. On February 13, 22 people became ill with gastroenteritis several hours after eating at a university cafeteria. Symptoms included nausea, vomiting, diarrhea, and abdominal cramps. Nine people were hospitalized. Canned mushrooms served with omelets and hamburgers were associated with illness. No deficiencies in food handling were found. Staphylococcal enterotoxin type A was identified in a sample of implicated mushrooms from the omelet bar and in unopened cans from the same lot.

Queens, New York. On February 28, 48 people became ill a median of 3 hours after eating lunch in a hospital employee cafeteria. One person was hospitalized. Canned mushrooms served at the salad bar were epidemiologically implicated. Two unopened cans of mushrooms from the same lot as the implicated can contained staphylococcal enterotoxin A.

McKeesport, Pennsylvania. On April 17, 12 people became ill with gastroenteritis a median of 2 hours after eating lunch or dinner at a restaurant. Two people were hospitalized. Canned mushrooms, consumed on pizza or with a parmigiana sauce, were associated with illness. No deficiencies were found in food preparation or storage. Staphylococcal enterotoxin was found in samples of remaining mushrooms and in unopened cans from the same lot.

Philipsburg, Pennsylvania. On April 22, 20 people developed illness several hours after eating food from a take-out pizzeria. Four people were hospitalized. Only pizza served with canned mushrooms was associated with illness. Staphylococcal enterotoxin was found in a sample of mushrooms from the pizzeria and in unopened cans with the same lot number.

For more information on recent outbreaks see the *Morbidity and Mortality Weekly Reports* from CDC.

12. Other Resources

A Loci index for genome *Staphylococcus aureus* is available from GenBank.

Campylobacter jejuni

1. Name of the Organism

Campylobacter jejuni (formerly known as *Campylobacter fetus* subsp. jejuni)

2. Name of Disease

Campylobacteriosis is the name of the illness caused by *C. jejuni*. It is also often known as campylobacter enteritis or gastroenteritis.

3. Major Symptoms

C. jejuni infection causes diarrhea, which may be watery or sticky and can contain blood (usually occult) and fecal leukocytes (white cells). Other symptoms often present are fever, abdominal pain, nausea, headache and muscle pain. The illness usually occurs 2–5 days after ingestion of the contaminated food or water. Illness generally lasts 7–10 days, but relapses are not uncommon (about 25% of cases). Most infections are self-limiting and are not treated with antibiotics. However, treatment with erythromycin does reduce the length of time that infected individuals shed the bacteria in their feces.

The infective dose of *C. jejuni* is considered to be small. Human feeding studies suggest that about 400–500 bacteria may cause illness in some individuals, while in others, greater numbers are required. A conducted volunteer human feeding study suggests that host susceptibility also dictates infectious dose to some degree. The pathogenic mechanisms of *C. jejuni* are still not completely understood, but it does produce a heat-labile toxin that may cause diarrhea. *C. jejuni* may also be an invasive organism.

4. Isolation Procedures

C. jejuni is usually present in high numbers in the diarrheal stools of individuals, but isolation requires special antibiotic-containing media and a special microaerophilic atmosphere (5% oxygen). However, most clinical laboratories are equipped to isolate *Campylobacter* spp. if requested.

5. Associated Foods

C. jejuni frequently contaminates raw chicken. Surveys show that 20 to 100% of retail chickens are contaminated. This is not overly surprising since many healthy chickens carry these bacteria in their intestinal tracts. Raw milk is also a source of infections. The bacteria are often carried by healthy cattle and by flies on farms. Non-chlorinated water may also be a source of infections. However, properly cooking chicken, pasteurizing milk, and chlorinating drinking water will kill the bacteria.

6. Frequency of the Disease

C. jejuni is the leading cause of bacterial diarrhea in the U.S. There are probably numbers of cases in excess of the estimated cases of salmonellosis (2- to 4,000,000/year).

7. Complications   Complications are relatively rare, but infections have been associated with reactive arthritis, hemolytic uremic syndrome, and following septicemia, infections of nearly any organ. The estimated case/fatality ratio for all *C. jejuni* infections is 0.1, meaning one death per 1,000 cases. Fatalities are rare in healthy individuals and usually occur in cancer patients or in the otherwise debilitated. Only 20 reported cases of septic abortion induced by *C. jejuni* have been recorded in the literature.

Meningitis, recurrent colitis, acute cholecystitis and Guillain-Barre syndrome are very rare complications.

8. Target Populations   Although anyone can have a *C. jejuni* infection, children under 5 years and young adults (15–29) are more frequently afflicted than other age groups. Reactive arthritis, a rare complication of these infections, is strongly associated with people who have the human lymphocyte antigen B27 (HLA-B27).

9. Recovery from Foods   Isolation of *C. jejuni* from food is difficult because the bacteria are usually present in very low numbers (unlike the case of diarrheal stools in which 10/6 bacteria/gram is not unusual). The methods require an enrichment broth containing antibiotics, special antibiotic-containing plates and a microaerophilic atmosphere generally with 5% oxygen and an elevated concentration of carbon dioxide (10%). Isolation can take several days to a week.

10. Selected Outbreaks   Usually outbreaks are small (less than 50 people), but in Bennington, VT, a large outbreak involving about 2,000 people occurred while the town was temporarily using a non-chlorinated water source as a water supply. Several small outbreaks have been reported among children who were taken on a class trip to a dairy and given raw milk to drink. An outbreak was also associated with consumption of raw clams. However, a survey showed that about 50% of infections are associated with either eating inadequately cooked or recontaminated chicken meat or handling chickens. It is the leading bacterial cause of sporadic (non-clustered cases) diarrheal disease in the U.S.

In April, 1986, an elementary school child was cultured for bacterial pathogens (due to bloody diarrhea), and *C. jejuni* was isolated. Food consumption/gastrointestinal illness questionnaires were administered to other students and faculty at the school. In all, 32 of 172 students reported symptoms of diarrhea (100%), cramps (80%), nausea (51%), fever (29%), vomiting (26%), and bloody stools (14%). The food questionnaire clearly implicated milk as the common source, and a dose/response was evident (those drinking more milk were more likely to be ill). Investigation of the dairy supplying the milk showed that they vat pasteurized the milk at 135 degrees F for 25 minutes rather than the required 145 degrees F for 30 minutes. The dairy processed surplus raw milk for the school, and this milk had a high somatic cell count. Cows from the herd supplying the dairy had *C. jejuni* in their feces. This outbreak points out the variation in symptoms which may occur with campylobacteriosis and the absolute need to adhere to pasteurization time/temperature standards.

Although other *Campylobacter* spp. have been implicated in human gastroenteritis (e.g., *C. laridis, C. hyointestinalis*), it is believed that 99% of the cases are caused by *C. jejuni.*

Information regarding an outbreak of *Campylobacter* in New Zealand is found in this MMWR 40(7):1991 Feb 22.

For more information on recent outbreaks see the *Morbidity and Mortality Weekly Reports* from CDC.

11. Education   The Food Safety Inspection Service of the U.S. Department of Agriculture has produced a background document on *Campylobacter.*

12. Other Resources   A Loci index for genome *Campylobacter jejuni* is available from GenBank.

Vibrio cholerae Serogroup O1

1. Name of the Organism   *Vibrio cholerae* Serogroup O1

2. Name of the Acute Disease   Cholera is the name of the infection caused by *V. cholerae.*

3. Nature of the Disease

Symptoms of Asiatic cholera may vary from a mild, watery diarrhea to an acute diarrhea, with characteristic rice water stools. Onset of the illness is generally sudden, with incubation periods varying from 6 hours to 5 days. Abdominal cramps, nausea, vomiting, dehydration, and shock; after severe fluid and electrolyte loss, death may occur. Illness is caused by the ingestion of viable bacteria, which attach to the small intestine and produce cholera toxin. The production of cholera toxin by the attached bacteria results in the watery diarrhea associated with this illness.

Infective dose—Human volunteer feeding studies utilizing healthy individuals have demonstrated that approximately one million organisms must be ingested to cause illness. Antacid consumption markedly lowers the infective dose.

4. Diagnosis of Human Illness

Cholera can be confirmed only by the isolation of the causative organism from the diarrheic stools of infected individuals.

5. Associated Foods

Cholera is generally a disease spread by poor sanitation, resulting in contaminated water supplies. This is clearly the main mechanism for the spread of cholera in poor communities in South America. The excellent sanitation facilities in the U.S. are responsible for the near eradication of epidemic cholera. Sporadic cases occur when shellfish harvested from fecally polluted coastal waters are consumed raw. Cholera may also be transmitted by shellfish harvested from nonpolluted waters since *V. cholerae* O1 is part of the autochthonous microbiota of these waters.

6. Frequency of Disease

Fewer than 80 proven cases of cholera have been reported in the U.S. since 1973. Most of these cases were detected only after epidemiological investigation. Probably more sporadic cases have occurred, but have gone undiagnosed or unreported.

7. The Usual Course of Disease and Some Complications

Individuals infected with cholera require rehydration either intravenously or orally with a solution containing sodium chloride, sodium bicarbonate, potassium chloride, and dextrose (glucose). The illness is generally self-limiting. Antibiotics such as tetracycline have been demonstrated to shorten the course of the illness. Death occurs from dehydration and loss of essential electrolytes. Medical treatment to prevent dehydration prevents all complications.

8. Target Populations

All people are believed to be susceptible to infection, but individuals with damaged or undeveloped immunity, reduced gastric acidity, or malnutrition may suffer more severe forms of the illness.

9. Analysis of Foods

V. cholerae serogroup O1 may be recovered from foods by methods similar to those used for recovering the organism from the feces of infected individuals. Pathogenic and nonpathogenic forms of the organism exist, so all food isolates must be tested for the production of cholera enterotoxin.

10. Selected Outbreaks

An incident of cholera in Indiana from imported food is reported in MMWR 44(20):1995 May 20.

See MMWR 44(11):1995 Mar 24 for an updated report on *Vibrio cholerae* O1 in the Western Hemisphere 1991–1994 and on *V. cholerae* O139 in Asia, 1994.

Surveillance for cholera in Cochabamba Department, Bolivia is discussed in this MMWR 42(33):1993 Aug 27.

The cholera outbreak in Burundi and Zimbabwe is detailed in the following MMWR 42(21):1993 Jun 04.

MMWR 40(49):1991 Dec 13 reports on a cholera outbreak associated with imported coconut milk.

A report of a cholera incident in New York is found in MMWR 40(30):1991 Aug 01.

Similar incidents in New Jersey and Florida are reported in MMWR 40(17):1991 May 03.

A case of importation of cholera from Peru to the United States is detailed in MMWR 40(15):1991 Apr 19.

The cholera outbreak in Peru is reported on in MMWR:40(6):1991 Feb 15, and the update of the South American endemic is in MMWR 40(13):1991 Apr 5.

For more information on recent outbreaks see the *Morbidity and Mortality Weekly Reports* from CDC.

11. Education

The CDC has a brochure on the prevention of cholera
- in English
- in Spanish
- in Portuguese

| **12. Other Resources** | A Loci index for genome *Vibrio cholerae* is available from GenBank. |

Listeria monocytogenes

| **1. Name of the Organism** | *Listeria monocytogenes* |

| **2. Name of Acute Disease** | Listeriosis is the name of the general group of disorders caused by *L. monocytogenes*. |

| **3. Nature of Disease** | Listeriosis is clinically defined when the organism is isolated from blood, cerebrospinal fluid, or an otherwise normally sterile site (e.g., placenta, fetus). |

The manifestations of listeriosis include septicemia, meningitis (or meningoencephalitis), encephalitis, and intrauterine or cervical infections in pregnant women, which may result in spontaneous abortion (2nd/3rd trimester) or stillbirth. The onset of the aforementioned disorders is usually preceded by influenza-like symptoms including persistent fever. It was reported that gastrointestinal symptoms such as nausea, vomiting, and diarrhea may precede more serious forms of listeriosis or may be the only symptoms expressed. Gastrointestinal symptoms were epidemiologically associated with use of antacids or cimetidine. The onset time to serious forms of listeriosis is unknown but may range from a few days to three weeks. The onset time to gastrointestinal symptoms is unknown but is probably greater than 12 hours.

The infective dose of *L. monocytogenes* is unknown but is believed to vary with the strain and susceptibility of the victim. From cases contracted through raw or supposedly pasteurized milk, it is safe to assume that in susceptible persons, fewer than 1,000 total organisms may cause disease. *L. monocytogenes* may invade the gastrointestinal epithelium. Once the bacterium enters the host's monocytes, macrophages, or polymorphonuclear leukocytes, it is bloodborne (septicemic) and can grow. Its presence intracellularly in phagocytic cells also permits access to the brain and probably transplacental migration to the fetus in pregnant women. The pathogenesis of *L. monocytogenes* centers on its ability to survive and multiply in phagocytic host cells.

4. Diagnosis of Human Illness Listeriosis can only be positively diagnosed by culturing the organism from blood, cerebrospinal fluid, or stool (although the latter is difficult and of limited value).

5. Associated Foods *L. monocytogenes* has been associated with such foods as raw milk, supposedly pasteurized fluid milk, cheeses (particularly soft-ripened varieties), ice cream, raw vegetables, fermented raw-meat sausages, raw and cooked poultry, raw meats (all types), and raw and smoked fish. Its ability to grow at temperatures as low as 3 degrees C permits multiplication in refrigerated foods.

6. Frequency of the Disease The 1987 incidence data prospectively collected by CDC suggests that there are at least 1600 cases of listeriosis with 415 deaths per year in the U.S. The vast majority of cases are sporadic, making epidemiological links to food very difficult.

7. Complications Most healthy persons probably show no symptoms. The "complications" are the usual clinical expressions of the disease.

When listeric meningitis occurs, the overall mortality may be as high as 70%; from septicemia 50%, from perinatal/neonatal infections greater than 80%. In infections during pregnancy, the mother usually survives. Successful treatment with parenteral penicillin or ampicillin has been reported. Trimethoprim-sulfamethoxazole has been shown effective in patients allergic to penicillin.

8. Target Populations The main target populations for listeriosis are:
- pregnant women/fetus—perinatal and neonatal infections;
- persons immunocompromised by corticosteroids, anticancer drugs, graft suppression therapy, AIDS;
- cancer patients—leukemic patients particularly;
- less frequently reported—diabetic, cirrhotic, asthmatic, and ulcerative colitis patients;
- the elderly;
- normal people—some reports suggest that normal, healthy people are at risk, although antacids or cimetidine may predispose. A listeriosis outbreak in Switzerland involving cheese suggested that healthy uncompromised

individuals could develop the disease, particularly if the foodstuff was heavily contaminated with the organism.

9. Food Analysis The methods for analysis of food are complex and time consuming. The present FDA method, revised in September, 1990, requires 24 and 48 hours of enrichment, followed by a variety of other tests. Total time to identification is from 5 to 7 days, but the announcement of specific nonradiolabeled DNA probes should soon allow a simpler and faster confirmation of suspect isolates.

Recombinant DNA technology may even permit 2–3 day positive analysis in the future. Currently, FDA is collaborating in adapting its methodology to quantify very low numbers of the organisms in foods.

10. Selected Outbreaks Outbreaks include the California episode in 1985, which was due to Mexican-style cheese and led to numerous stillbirths. As a result of this episode, FDA has been monitoring domestic and imported cheeses and has taken numerous actions to remove these products from the market when *L. monocytogenes* is found.

There have been other clustered cases, such as in Philadelphia, PA, in 1987. Specific food linkages were only made epidemiologically in this cluster.

CDC has established an epidemiological link between consumption of raw hot dogs or undercooked chicken and approximately 20% of the sporadic cases under prospective study.

For more information on recent outbreaks see the *Morbidity and Mortality Weekly Reports* from CDC.

11. Education The FDA health alert for Hispanic pregnant women concerns the risk of listeriosis from soft cheeses. The CDC provides similar information in Spanish.

The Food Safety and Inspection Service of the U.S. Department of Agriculture has jointly produced with the FDA a background document on Listeria and Listeriosis. FSIS also has updated consumer information on Listeria dated February 1999.

The CDC produces an information brochure on preventing Listeriosis.

12. Other Resources A Loci index for genome *Listeria monocytogenes* is available from GenBank.

Clostridium perfringens

1. Name of Organism

Clostridium perfringens

2. Name of Acute Disease

Perfringens food poisoning is the term used to describe the common foodborne illness caused by C. perfringens. A more serious but rare illness is also caused by ingesting food contaminated with Type C strains. The latter illness is known as enteritis necroticans or pig-bel disease.

3. Nature of Disease

The common form of perfringens poisoning is characterized by intense abdominal cramps and diarrhea which begin 8–22 hours after consumption of foods containing large numbers of those C. perfringens bacteria capable of producing the food poisoning toxin. The illness is usually over within 24 hours but less severe symptoms may persist in some individuals for 1 or 2 weeks. A few deaths have been reported as a result of dehydration and complications.

Necrotic enteritis (pig-bel) caused by C. perfringens is often fatal. This disease also begins as a result of ingesting large numbers of the causative bacteria in contaminated foods. Deaths from necrotic enteritis (pig-bel syndrome) are caused by infection and necrosis of the intestines and from resulting septicemia. This disease is very rare in the U.S.

Infective dose—The symptoms are caused by ingestion of large numbers (greater than 10 to the 8th) vegetative cells. Toxin production in the digestive tract (or in test tubes) is associated with sporulation. This disease is a food infection; only one episode has ever implied the possibility of intoxication (i.e., disease from preformed toxin).

4. Diagnosis of Human Illness

Perfringens poisoning is diagnosed by its symptoms and the typical delayed onset of illness. Diagnosis is confirmed by detecting the toxin in the feces of patients. Bacteriological confirmation can also be done by finding exceptionally large numbers of the causative bacteria in implicated foods or in the feces of patients.

5. Associated Foods and Food Handling

In most instances, the actual cause of poisoning by C. perfringens is temperature abuse of prepared foods. Small numbers of the organisms are often present after cooking and multiply to food poisoning levels during cool down and storage of prepared foods. Meats, meat products, and gravy are the foods most frequently implicated.

6. Frequency

Perfringens poisoning is one of the most commonly reported foodborne illnesses in the U.S. There were 1,162 cases in 1981, in 28 separate outbreaks. At least 10–20 outbreaks have been reported annually in the U.S. for the past 2 decades. Typically, dozens or even hundreds of person are affected. It is probable that many outbreaks go unreported because the implicated foods or patient feces are not tested routinely for *C. perfringens* or its toxin. CDC estimates that about 10,000 actual cases occur annually in the U.S.

7. Usual Course of Disease and Complications

The disease generally lasts 24 hours. In the elderly or infirm, symptoms may last 1–2 weeks. Complications and/or death only very rarely occur.

8. Target Populations

Institutional feeding (such as school cafeterias, hospitals, nursing homes, prisons, etc.) where large quantities of food are prepared several hours before serving is the most common circumstance in which perfringens poisoning occurs. The young and elderly are the most frequent victims of perfringens poisoning. Except in the case of pig-bel syndrome, complications are few in persons under 30 years of age. Elderly persons are more likely to experience prolonged or severe symptoms.

9. Analysis of Food and Feces

Standard bacteriological culturing procedures are used to detect the organism in implicated foods and in feces of patients. Serological assays are used for detecting enterotoxin in the feces of patients and for testing the ability of strains to produce toxin. The procedures take 1–3 days.

10. Selected Outbreaks

Since December 1981, FDA has investigated 10 outbreaks in 5 states. In two instances, more than one outbreak occurred in the same feeding facility within a 3-week period. One such outbreak occurred on 19 March 1984, involving 77 prison inmates. Roast beef served as a luncheon meat was implicated as the food vehicle and *C. perfringens* was confirmed as the cause by examining stools of 24 patients. Most of the patients became ill 8–16 hours after the meal. Eight days later, on 27 March 1984, a second outbreak occurred involving many of the same persons. The food vehicle was ham. Inadequate refrigeration and insufficient reheating of the implicated foods caused the outbreaks. Most of the other outbreaks occurred in institutional feeding environments: a hospital, nursing home, labor camp, school cafeteria, and at a fire house luncheon.

In November, 1985, a large outbreak of C. *perfringens* gastroenteritis occurred among factory workers in Connecticut. Forty-four percent of the 1,362 employees were affected. Four main-course foods served at an employee banquet were associated with illness, but gravy was implicated by stratified analysis. The gravy had been prepared 12–24 hours before serving, had been improperly cooled, and was reheated shortly before serving. The longer the reheating period, the less likely the gravy was to cause illness.

A outbreak of C. *perfringens* in corned beef was reported in MMWR 43(8):1994 Mar 04.

For more information on recent outbreaks see the *Morbidity and Mortality Weekly Reports* from CDC.

Bacillus cereus and Other *Bacillus* spp.

1. Name of the Organism
Bacillus cereus and other *Bacillus* spp.

Bacillus cereus is a Gram-positive, facultatively aerobic sporeformer whose cells are large rods and whose spores do not swell the sporangium. These and other characteristics, including biochemical features, are used to differentiate and confirm the presence of B. *cereus*, although these characteristics are shared with B. *cereus* var. mycoides, B. *thuringiensis* and B. *anthracis*. Differentiation of these organisms depends upon determination of motility (most B. *cereus* are motile), presence of toxin crystals (B. *thuringiensis*), hemolytic activity (B. *cereus* and others are beta hemolytic whereas B. *anthracis* is usually nonhemolytic), and rhizoid growth which is characteristic of B. *cereus* var. mycoides.

2. Name of Illness
B. *cereus* food poisoning is the general description, although two recognized types of illness are caused by two distinct metabolites. The diarrheal type of illness is caused by a large molecular weight protein,

while the vomiting (emetic) type of illness is believed to be caused by a low molecular weight, heat-stable peptide.

3. Nature of Illness

The symptoms of B. cereus diarrheal type food poisoning mimic those of Clostridium perfringens food poisoning. The onset of watery diarrhea, abdominal cramps, and pain occurs 6–15 hours after consumption of contaminated food. Nausea may accompany diarrhea, but vomiting (emesis) rarely occurs. Symptoms persist for 24 hours in most instances.

The emetic type of food poisoning is characterized by nausea and vomiting within 0.5 to 6 hours after consumption of contaminated foods. Occasionally, abdominal cramps and/or diarrhea may also occur. Duration of symptoms is generally less than 24 hours. The symptoms of this type of food poisoning parallel those caused by Staphylococcus aureus foodborne intoxication. Some strains of B. subtilis and B. licheniformis have been isolated from lamb and chicken incriminated in food poisoning episodes. These organisms demonstrate the production of a highly heat-stable toxin which may be similar to the vomiting type toxin produced by B. cereus.

The presence of large numbers of B. cereus (greater than 10^6 organisms/g) in a food is indicative of active growth and proliferation of the organism and is consistent with a potential hazard to health.

4. Diagnosis of Human Illness

Confirmation of B. cereus as the etiologic agent in a foodborne outbreak requires either (1) isolation of strains of the same serotype from the suspect food and feces or vomitus of the patient, (2) isolation of large numbers of a B. cereus serotype known to cause foodborne illness from the suspect food or from the feces or vomitus of the patient, or (3) isolation of B. cereus from suspect foods and determining their enterotoxigenicity by serological (diarrheal toxin) or biological (diarrheal and emetic) tests. The rapid onset time to symptoms in the emetic form of disease, coupled with some food evidence, is often sufficient to diagnose this type of food poisoning.

5. Foods Incriminated

A wide variety of foods including meats, milk, vegetables, and fish have been associated with the diarrheal type food poisoning. The vomiting-type outbreaks have generally been associated with rice products; however, other starchy foods such as potato, pasta and cheese products have also been implicated. Food mixtures such as sauces, puddings, soups, casseroles, pastries, and salads have frequently been incriminated in food poisoning outbreaks.

6. Relative Frequency of Illness

In 1980, 9 outbreaks were reported to the Centers for Disease Control and included such foods as beef, turkey, and Mexican foods. In 1981, 8 outbreaks were reported which primarily involved rice and shellfish. Other outbreaks go unreported or are misdiagnosed because of symptomatic similarities to *Staphylococcus aureus* intoxication (*B. cereus* vomiting-type) or *C. perfringens* food poisoning (*B. cereus* diarrheal type).

7. Complications

Although no specific complications have been associated with the diarrheal and vomiting toxins produced by *B. cereus*, other clinical manifestations of *B. cereus* invasion or contamination have been observed. They include bovine mastitis, severe systemic and pyogenic infections, gangrene, septic meningitis, cellulitis, panophthalmitis, lung abscesses, infant death, and endocarditis.

8. Target Populations

All people are believed to be susceptible to *B. cereus* food poisoning.

9. Food Analysis

A variety of methods have been recommended for the recovery, enumeration and confirmation of *B. cereus* in foods. More recently, a serological method has been developed for detecting the putative enterotoxin of *B. cereus* (diarrheal type) isolates from suspect foods. Recent investigations suggest that the vomiting type toxin can be detected by animal models (cats, monkeys) or possibly by cell culture.

10. Selected Outbreaks

On September 22, 1985, the Maine Bureau of Health was notified of gastrointestinal illness among patrons of a Japanese restaurant. Because the customers were exhibiting symptoms of illness while still on the restaurant premises, and because uncertainty existed as to the etiology of the problem, the local health department, in concurrence with the restaurant owner, closed the restaurant at 7:30 P.M. that same day.

Eleven (31%) of the approximately 36 patrons reportedly served on the evening of September 22 were contacted in an effort to determine the etiology of the outbreak. Those 11 comprised the last three dining parties served on September 22. Despite extensive publicity, no additional cases were reported.

A case was defined as anyone who demonstrated vomiting or diarrhea within 6 hours of dining at the restaurant. All 11 individuals were interviewed for symptoms, time of onset of illness, illness duration, and foods ingested. All 11 reported nausea and vomiting; nine reported diarrhea; one reported headache; and one reported abdominal cramps. Onset of illness ranged from 30 minutes to 5 hours (mean 1 hour, 23 minutes) after eating at the restaurant. Duration of illness ranged from 5 hours to several days, except for two individuals still symptomatic with diarrhea 2 weeks after dining at the restaurant. Ten persons sought medical treatment at local emergency rooms on September 22; two ultimately required hospitalization for rehydration.

Analysis of the association of specific foods with illness was not instructive, since all persons consumed the same food items; chicken soup, fried shrimp, stir-fried rice, fried zucchini, onions, bean sprouts, cucumber, cabbage, and lettuce salad, ginger salad dressing, hibachi chicken and steak, and tea. Five persons ordered hibachi scallops, and one person ordered hibachi swordfish. However, most individuals sampled each other's entrees. One vomitus specimen and two stool specimens from the three separate individuals yielded an overgrowth of *B. cereus*, although an accurate bacterial count could not be made because an inadequate amount of the steak remained for laboratory analysis. No growth of *B. cereus* was reported from the fried rice, mixed fried vegetables, or hibachi chicken.

According to the owner, all meat was delivered 2–3 times a week from a local meat supplier and refrigerated until ordered by restaurant patrons. Appropriate-sized portions for a dining group were taken from the kitchen to the dining area and diced or sliced, then sauteed at the table directly in front of restaurant patrons. The meat was seasoned with soy sauce, salt and white pepper, open containers of which had been used for at least 2 months by the restaurant. The hibachi steak was served immediately after cooking.

The fried rice served with the meal was customarily made from leftover boiled rice. It could not be established whether the boiled rice had been stored refrigerated or at room temperature.

Fresh, rapidly cooked meat, eaten immediately, seems an unlikely vehicle of *B. cereus* food poisoning. The laboratory finding of *B. cereus* in a foodstuff without quantitative cultures and without accompanying epidemiologic data is insufficient to establish its role in the outbreak. Although no viable *B. cereus* organisms were isolated from the fried rice eaten with the meal, it does not exclude this food as the common vehicle. Reheating during preparation may have eliminated the bacteria in the food without decreasing the activity of the heat-stable toxin. While the question of the specific vehicle remains incompletely resolved, the clinical and laboratory findings substantially support *B. cereus* as the cause of the outbreak.

Most episodes of food poisoning undoubtedly go unreported, and in most of those reported, the specific pathogens are never identified. Alert recognition of the clinical syndrome and appropriate laboratory work permitted identification of the role of *B. cereus* in this outbreak.

For a report on a *B. cereus* outbreak in northern Virginia see this MMWR 43(10):1994 Mar 18.

For more information on recent outbreaks see the *Morbidity and Mortality Weekly Reports* from CDC.

Enteropathogenic *Escherichia coli*

1. Name of the Organism   Enteropathogenic *Escherichia coli* (EPEC)

Currently, there are four recognized classes of enterovirulent *E. coli* (collectively referred to as the EEC group) that cause gastroenteritis in humans. Among these are the enteropathogenic (EPEC) strains. EPEC are defined as *E. coli* belonging to serogroups epidemiologically implicated as pathogens but whose virulence mechanism is unrelated to the excretion of typical *E. coli* enterotoxins. *E. coli* are Gram-negative, rod-shaped bacteria belonging to the family Enterobacteriaceae. Source(s) and prevalence of EPEC are controversial because foodborne outbreaks are sporadic. Humans, bovines, and swine can be infected, and the latter often serve as common experimental animal models. *E. coli* are present in the normal gut flora of these mammals. The proportion of pathogenic to nonpathogenic strains, although the subject of intense research, is unknown.

2. Name of Acute Disease

Infantile diarrhea is the name of the disease usually associated with EPEC.

3. Nature of Disease

EPEC causes either a watery or bloody diarrhea, the former associated with the attachment to, and physical alteration of, the integrity of the intestine. Bloody diarrhea is associated with attachment and an acute tissue-destructive process, perhaps caused by a toxin similar to that of *Shigella dysenteriae*, also called verotoxin. In most of these strains the shiga-like toxin is cell-associated rather than excreted.

Infective dose—EPEC are highly infectious for infants and the dose is presumably very low. In the few documented cases of adult diseases, the dose is presumably similar to other colonizers (greater than 10^6 total dose).

4. Diagnosis of Human Illness

The distinction of EPEC from other groups of pathogenic *E. coli* isolated from patients' stools involves serological and cell culture assays. Serotyping, although useful, is not strict for EPEC.

5. Associated Foods

Common foods implicated in EPEC outbreaks are raw beef and chicken, although any food exposed to fecal contamination is strongly suspect.

6. Relative Frequency of Disease

Outbreaks of EPEC are sporadic. Incidence varies on a worldwide basis; countries with poor sanitation practices have the most frequent outbreaks.

7. Usual Course of Disease and Some Complications

Occasionally, diarrhea in infants is prolonged, leading to dehydration, electrolyte imbalance and death (50% mortality rates have been reported in third world countries).

8. Target Populations

EPEC outbreaks most often affect infants, especially those that are bottle fed, suggesting that contaminated water is often used to rehydrate infant formulae in underdeveloped countries.

9. Analysis of Foods

The isolation and identification of *E. coli* in foods follows standard enrichment and biochemical procedures. Serotyping of isolates to distinguish EPEC is laborious and requires high quality, specific antisera, and technical expertise. The total analysis may require from 7 to 14 days.

10. Selected Outbreaks

Sporadic outbreaks of EPEC diarrhea have occurred for half a century in infant nurseries, presumably derived from the hospital environment or contaminated infant formula. Common-source outbreaks of EPEC diarrhea involving healthy young adults were reported in the late 1960s. Presumably a large inoculum was ingested.

For more information on recent outbreaks see the *Morbidity and Mortality Weekly Reports* from CDC.

Escherichia coli O157:H7

1. Name of the Organism

Escherichia coli O157:H7 (enterohemorrhagic *E. coli* or EHEC)

Currently, there are four recognized classes of enterovirulent *E. coli* (collectively referred to as the EEC group) that cause gastroenteritis in humans. Among these is the enterohemorrhagic (EHEC) strain designated *E. coli* O157:H7. *E. coli* is a normal inhabitant of the intestines of all animals, including humans. When aerobic culture methods are used, *E. coli* is the dominant species found in feces. Normally *E. coli* serves a useful function in the body by suppressing the growth of harmful bacterial species and by synthesizing appreciable amounts of vitamins. A minority *of E. coli* strains are capable of causing human illness by several different mechanisms. *E. coli* serotype O157:H7 is a rare variety of *E. coli* that produces large quantities of one or more related, potent toxins that cause severe damage to the lining of the intestine. These toxins (verotoxin [VT], shiga-like toxin) are closely related or identical to the toxin produced by *Shigella dysenteriae*.

2. Name of Acute Disease

Hemorrhagic colitis is the name of the acute disease caused by *E. coli* O157:H7.

3. Nature of Disease

The illness is characterized by severe cramping (abdominal pain) and diarrhea which is initially watery but becomes grossly bloody. Occasionally vomiting occurs. Fever is either low-grade or absent. The illness is usually self-limited and lasts for an average of 8 days. Some individuals exhibit watery diarrhea only.

Infective dose—Unknown, but from a compilation of outbreak data, including the organism's ability to be passed person-to-person in the day-care setting and nursing homes, the dose may be similar to that of *Shigella* spp. (10 organisms).

4. Diagnosis of Human Illness

Hemorrhagic colitis is diagnosed by isolation of *E. coli* of serotype O157:H7 or other verotoxin-producing *E. coli* from diarrheal stools. Alternatively, the stools can be tested directly for the presence of verotoxin. Confirmation can be obtained by isolation of *E. coli* of the same serotype from the incriminated food.

5. Associated Foods

Undercooked or raw hamburger (ground beef) has been implicated in nearly all documented outbreaks and in other sporadic cases. Raw milk was the vehicle in a school outbreak in Canada. These are the only two demonstrated food causes of disease, but other meats may contain *E. coli* O157:H7.

6. Relative Frequency of Disease

Hemorrhagic colitis infections are not too common, but this is probably not reflective of the true frequency. In the Pacific Northwest, *E. coli* O157:H7 is thought to be second only to Salmonella as a cause of bacterial diarrhea. Because of the unmistakable symptoms of profuse, visible blood in severe cases, those victims probably seek medical attention, but less severe cases are probably more numerous.

7. Usual Course of Disease and Some Complications

Some victims, particularly the very young, have developed hemolytic uremic syndrome (HUS), characterized by renal failure and hemolytic anemia. From 0 to 15% of hemorrhagic colitis victims may develop HUS. The disease can lead to permanent loss of kidney function.

In the elderly, HUS, plus two other symptoms, fever and neurologic symptoms, constitutes thrombotic thrombocytopenic purpura (TTP). This illness can have a mortality rate in the elderly as high as 50%.

8. Target Populations

All people are believed to be susceptible to hemorrhagic colitis, but larger outbreaks have occurred in institutional settings.

9. Analysis of Foods

E. coli O157:H7 will form colonies on agar media that are selective for *E. coli*. However, the high temperature growth procedure normally performed to eliminate background organisms before plating cannot be used because of the inability of these organisms to grow at temperatures of 44.0–45.5 degrees C that support the growth of most *E. coli*. The use of DNA probes to detect genes encoding for the production of verotoxins (VT1 and VT2) is the most sensitive method devised.

10. Selected Outbreaks

Three outbreaks occurred in 1982. Two of them, one in Michigan and one in Oregon, involved hamburgers from a national fast-food chain. The third occurred in a home for the aged in Ottawa, Ontario; club sandwiches were implicated, and 19 people died. More recently, several outbreaks in nursing homes and a day-care center have been investigated. Two large outbreaks occurred in 1984, one in 1985, three in 1986. Larger outbreaks have occurred in the Northwest U.S. and Canada.

In October-November, 1986, an outbreak of hemorrhagic colitis caused by *E. coli* O157:H7 occurred in Walla Walla, WA. Thirty-seven people, aged 11 months to 78 years developed diarrhea caused by the organism. All isolates from patients (14) had a unique plasmid profile and produced Shiga-like toxin II. In addition to diarrhea, 36 persons reported grossly bloody stools and 36 of the 37 reported abdominal cramps. Seventeen patients were hospitalized. One patient developed HUS (4 years old) and three developed TTP (70, 78, and 78 years old). Two patients with TTP died. Ground beef was the implicated food vehicle.

An excellent summary of nine *E. coli* O157:H7 outbreaks appeared in the Annals of Internal Medicine, 1 November, 1988, pp. 705–712.

There was a recall of frozen hamburger underway (12 Aug 1997). For more information, see the USDA announcement and follow-up announcement (15 Aug 1997) on the U.S. Department of Agriculture web site concerning the recall of Hudson frozen ground beef.

The Centers for Disease Control and Prevention have reported on the above outbreak in preliminary

(MMWR 45(44):975, 1996 November 8) and in up-dated (MMWR 46(1):4–8, 1997 January 10) form.

The FDA has issued on 31 October 1996 a press release concerning an outbreak of *E. coli* O157:H7 associated with Odwalla brand apple juice products.

A non-food related outbreak of *E. coli* O157:H7 is reported in MMWR 45(21):1996 May 31. While the source of the outbreak is thought to be waterborne, the article is linked to this chapter to provide up-dated reference information on enterohemorrhagic *E. coli*.

MMWR 45(12):1996 Mar 29 reports on an outbreak of O157:H7 that occurred in Georgia and Tennessee in June of 1995.

A community outbreak of hemolytic uremic syndrome attributable to *Escherichia coli* O111:NM in southern Australia in 1995 is reported in MMWR 44(29):1995 Jul 28.

A report on enhanced detection of sporadic *E. coli* O157:H7 infections in New Jersey and on an *E. coli* O157:H7 outbreak at a summer camp are in MMWR 44(22):1995 Jun 9.

An outbreak of *E. coli* O157:H7 in Washington and California associated with dry-cured salami is re-ported in MMWR 44(9):1995 Mar 10.

Information concerning an outbreak that occurred because of home-cooked hamburger can be found in this MMWR 43(12):1994 Apr 01.

MMWR 43(10):1994 Mar 18 reports on laboratory screening for *E. coli* O157 in Connecticut.

The outbreak of EHEC in the western states of the US is reported in preliminary form in this MMWR 42(4):1993 Feb 5, and in updated form in this MMWR 42(14):1993 Apr 16.

An outbreak of *E. coli* O157 in 1990 in North Dakota is reported in the MMWR 40(16):1991 Apr 26.

The Centers for Disease Control and Prevention has reissued the 5 November 1982 MMWR report that was the first to describe the diarrheal illness of *E. coli* O157:H7. This reissue is a part of the com-memoration of CDC's 50th anniversary.

For more information on recent outbreaks see the *Morbidity and Mortality Weekly Reports* from CDC.

11. Education USDA Urges Consumers To Use Food Thermometer When Cooking Ground Beef Patties (Aug 11 1998)

The CDC has an information brochure on preventing *Escherichia coli* O157:H7 infections.

12. Other Resources

Dr. Feng of FDA/CFSAN has written a monograph on *E. coli* O157:H7 which appeared in the CDC journal Emerging Infectious Diseases Vol. 1 No. 2, April-June 1995.

Enteroinvasive *Escherichia coli*

1. Name of the Organism

Enteroinvasive *Escherichia coli* or (EIEC)

Currently, there are four recognized classes of enterovirulent *E. coli* (collectively referred to as the EEC group) that cause gastroenteritis in humans. *E. coli* is part of the normal intestinal flora of humans and other primates. A minority of *E. coli* strains are capable of causing human illness by several different mechanisms. Among these are the enteroinvasive (EIEC) strains. It is unknown what foods may harbor these pathogenic enteroinvasive (EIEC) strains responsible for a form of bacillary dysentery.

2. Name of Disease

Enteroinvasive *E. coli* (EIEC) may produce an illness known as bacillary dysentery. The EIEC strains responsible for this syndrome are closely related to *Shigella* spp.

3. Nature of the Disease

Following the ingestion of EIEC, the organisms invade the epithelial cells of the intestine, resulting in a mild form of dysentery, often mistaken for dysentery caused by *Shigella* species. The illness is characterized by the appearance of blood and mucus in the stools of infected individuals.

Infective dose—The infectious dose of EIEC is thought to be as few as 10 organisms (same as *Shigella*).

4. Diagnosis of Human Illness

The culturing of the organism from the stools of infected individuals and the demonstration of invasiveness of isolates in tissue culture or in a suitable animal model is necessary to diagnose dysentery caused by this organism.

More recently, genetic probes for the invasiveness genes of both EIEC and *Shigella* spp. have been developed.

5. Associated Foods

It is currently unknown what foods may harbor EIEC, but any food contaminated with human feces from an ill individual, either directly or via contaminated water, could cause disease in others. Outbreaks have been associated with hamburger meat and unpasteurized milk.

6. Relative Frequency of Disease

One major foodborne outbreak attributed to enteroinvasive *E. coli* in the U.S. occurred in 1973. It was due to the consumption of imported cheese from France. The disease caused by EIEC is uncommon, but it may be confused with shigellosis and its prevalence may be underestimated.

7. The Usual Course of Disease and Some Complications

Dysentery caused by EIEC usually occurs within 12 to 72 hours following the ingestion of contaminated food. The illness is characterized by abdominal cramps, diarrhea, vomiting, fever, chills, and a generalized malaise. Dysentery caused by this organism is generally self-limiting with no known complications. A common sequelus associated with infection, especially in pediatric cases, is hemolytic uremic syndrome (HUS).

8. Target Populations

All people are subject to infection by this organism.

9. Analysis of Foods

Foods are examined as are stool cultures. Detection of this organism in foods is extremely difficult because undetectable levels may cause illness. It is estimated that the ingestion of as few as 10 organisms may result in dysentery.

10. Selected Outbreaks

Several outbreaks in the U.S. have been attributed to this organism. One outbreak occurred in 1973 and was due to the consumption of imported cheese. More recently, a cruise ship outbreak was attributed to potato salad, and an outbreak occurred in a home for the mentally retarded where subsequent person-to-person transmission occurred.

For more information on recent outbreaks see the *Morbidity and Mortality Weekly Reports* from CDC.

Shigella spp.

1. Name of the Organism

Shigella spp. (*Shigella sonnei, S. boydii, S. flexneri,* and *S. dysenteriae*)

Shigella are Gram-negative, nonmotile, nonspore-forming rod-shaped bacteria. The illness caused by *Shigella* (shigellosis) accounts for less than 10% of the reported outbreaks of foodborne illness in this country. *Shigella* rarely occurs in animals; principally a disease of humans except other primates such as monkeys and chimpanzees. The organism is frequently found in water polluted with human feces.

2. Name of Disease

Shigellosis (bacillary dysentery).

3. Nature of Disease

Symptoms—Abdominal pain; cramps; diarrhea; fever; vomiting; blood, pus, or mucus in stools; tenesmus.

Onset time—12 to 50 hours.

Infective dose—As few as 10 cells depending on age and condition of host. The *Shigella* spp. are highly infectious agents that are transmitted by the fecal-oral route.

The disease is caused when virulent *Shigella* organisms attach to, and penetrate, epithelial cells of the intestinal mucosa. After invasion, they multiply intracellularly, and spread to contiguous epitheleal cells resulting in tissue destruction. Some strains produce enterotoxin and Shiga toxin (very much like the verotoxin of *E. coli* O157:H7).

4. Diagnosis of Human Illness

Serological identification of culture isolated from stool.

5. Associated Foods

Salads (potato, tuna, shrimp, macaroni, and chicken), raw vegetables, milk and dairy products, and poultry. Contamination of these foods is usually through the fecal-oral route. Fecally contaminated water and unsanitary handling by food handlers are the most common causes of contamination.

6. Relative Frequency of Disease

An estimated 300,000 cases of shigellosis occur annually in the U.S. The number attributable to food is unknown, but given the low infectious dose, it is probably substantial.

7. Complications

Infections are associated with mucosal ulceration, rectal bleeding, drastic dehydration; fatality may be as high as 10–15% with some strains. Reiter's disease, reactive arthritis, and hemolytic uremic syndrome are possible sequelae that have been reported in the aftermath of shigellosis.

8. Target Populations

Infants, the elderly, and the infirm are susceptible to the severest symptoms of disease, but all humans are susceptible to some degree. Shigellosis is a very common malady suffered by individuals with acquired immune deficiency syndrome (AIDS) and AIDS-related complex, as well as non-AIDS homosexual men.

9. Food Analysis Organisms are difficult to demonstrate in foods because methods are not developed or are insensitive. A genetic probe to the virulence plasmid has been developed by FDA and is currently under field test. However, the isolation procedures are still poor.

10. Selected Outbreaks In 1985, a huge outbreak of foodborne shigellosis occurred in Midland-Odessa, Texas, involving perhaps as many as 5,000 persons. The implicated food was chopped, bagged lettuce, prepared in a central location for a Mexican restaurant chain. FDA research subsequently showed that *S. sonnei,* the isolate from the lettuce, could survive in chopped lettuce under refrigeration, and the lettuce remained fresh and appeared to be quite edible.

In 1985–1986, several outbreaks of shigellosis occurred on college campuses, usually associated with fresh vegetables from the salad bar. Usually an ill food service worker was shown to be the cause.

In 1987, several very large outbreaks of shigellosis *(S. sonnei)* occurred involving thousands of persons, but no specific food vector could be proven.

In 1988, numerous individuals contracted shigellosis from food consumed aboard Northwest Airlines flights; food on these flights had been prepared in one central commissary. No specific food item was implicated, but various sandwiches were suspected.

Note: Although all *Shigella* spp. have been implicated in foodborne outbreaks at some time, *S. sonnei* is clearly the leading cause of shigellosis from food. The other species are more closely associated with contaminated water. One in particular, *S. flexneri,* is now thought to be in large part sexually transmitted.

For information on the outbreak of *Shigella* on a cruise ship, see MMWR 43(35):1994 Sep 09.

MMWR 40(25):1991 Jun 28 reports on a *Shigella dysenteriae* Type 1 outbreak in Guatemala, 1991.

For more information on recent outbreaks see the *Morbidity and Mortality Weekly Reports* from CDC.

Miscellaneous Enterics

1. Name of the Organism

Miscellaneous enterics, Gram-negative genera including: *Klebsiella, Enterobacter, Proteus, Citrobacter, Aerobacter, Providencia, Serratia*

2. Name of Acute Disease

Gastroenteritis is name of the disease occasionally and sporadically caused by these genera.

3. Nature of Disease

Acute gastroenteritis is characterized by two or more of the symptoms of vomiting, nausea, fever, chills, abdominal pain, and watery (dehydrating) diarrhea occurring 12–24 hours after ingestion of contaminated food or water. Chronic diarrheal disease is characterized by dysenteric symptoms: foul-smelling, mucus-containing, diarrheic stool with flatulence and abdominal distention. The chronic disease may continue for months and require antibiotic treatment.

Infectious dose—unknown. Both the acute and chronic forms of the disease are suspected to result from the elaboration of enterotoxins. These organisms may become transiently virulent by gaining mobilizeable genetic elements from other pathogens. For example, pathogenic *Citrobacter freundii* which elaborated a toxin identical to *E. coli* heat-stable toxin was isolated from the stools of ill children.

4. Diagnosis of Human Illness

Recovery and identification methods for these organisms from food, water or diarrheal specimens are based upon the efficacy of selective media and results of microbiological and biochemical assays. The ability to produce enterotoxin(s) may be determined by cell culture assay and animal bioassays, serological methods, or genetic probes.

5. Associated Foods

These bacteria have been recovered from dairy products, raw shellfish, and fresh raw vegetables. The organisms occur in soils used for crop production and shellfish harvesting waters and, therefore, may pose a health hazard.

6. Relative Frequency of Disease

Acute gastrointestinal illness may occur more frequently in undeveloped areas of the world. The chronic illness is common in malnourished children living in unsanitary conditions in tropical countries.

7. Usual Course of Disease

Healthy individuals recover quickly and without treatment from the acute form of gastrointestinal

and Some Complications disease. Malnourished children (1–4 years) and infants who endure chronic diarrhea soon develop structural and functional abnormalities of their intestinal tracts resulting in loss of ability to absorb nutrients. Death is not uncommon in these children and results indirectly from the chronic toxigenic effects which produce the malabsorption and malnutrition.

8. Target Populations All people may be susceptible to pathogenic forms of these bacteria. Protracted illness is more commonly experienced by the very young.

9. Food Analysis These strains are recovered by standard selective and differential isolation procedures for enteric bacteria. Biochemical and in vitro assays may be used to determine species and pathogenic potential. Not being usually thought of as human pathogens, they may easily be overlooked by the clinical microbiology laboratory.

10. Selected Outbreaks Intestinal infections with these species in the U.S. have usually taken the form of sporadic cases of somewhat doubtful etiology.

Citrobacter freundii was suspected by CDC of causing an outbreak of diarrheal disease in Washington, DC. Imported Camembert cheese was incriminated.

For more information on recent outbreaks see the *Morbidity and Mortality Weekly Reports* from CDC.

Streptococcus spp.

1. Name of the Organism *Streptococcus*

The genus *Streptococcus* is comprised of Gram-positive, *microaerophilic cocci* (round), which are not motile and occur in chains or pairs. The genus is defined by a combination of antigenic, hemolytic, and physiological characteristics into Groups A, B, C, D, F, and G. Groups A and D can be transmitted to humans via food.

Group A: one species with 40 antigenic types *(S. pyogenes)*.

Group D: five species *(S. faecalis, S. faecium, S. durans, S. avium,* and *S. bovis)*.

2. Name of Acute Disease Group A: Cause septic sore throat and scarlet fever as well as other pyogenic and septicemic infections.

Group D: May produce a clinical syndrome similar to staphylococcal intoxication.

3. Nature of Illness/ Disease

Group A: Sore and red throat, pain on swallowing, tonsilitis, high fever, headache, nausea, vomiting, malaise, rhinorrhea; occasionally a rash occurs, onset 1–3 days; the infectious dose is probably quite low (less than 1,000 organisms).

Group D: Diarrhea, abdominal cramps, nausea, vomiting, fever, chills, dizziness in 2–36 hours. Following ingestion of suspect food, the infectious dose is probably high (greater than 107 organisms).

4. Diagnosis of Human Disease

Group A: Culturing of nasal and throat swabs, pus, sputum, blood, suspect food, environmental samples.

Group D: Culturing of stool samples, blood, and suspect food.

5. Associated Foods

Group A: Food sources include milk, ice cream, eggs, steamed lobster, ground ham, potato salad, egg salad, custard, rice pudding, and shrimp salad. In almost all cases, the foodstuffs were allowed to stand at room temperature for several hours between preparation and consumption. Entrance into the food is the result of poor hygiene, ill food handlers, or the use of unpasteurized milk.

Group D: Food sources include sausage, evaporated milk, cheese, meat croquettes, meat pie, pudding, raw milk, and pasteurized milk. Entrance into the food chain is due to underprocessing and/or poor and unsanitary food preparation.

6. Relative Frequency of Infection

Group A infections are low and may occur in any season, whereas Group D infections are variable.

7. Usual Course of Disease and Complications

Group A: Streptococcal sore throat is very common, especially in children. Usually it is successfully treated with antibiotics. Complications are rare and the fatality rate is low.

Group D: Diarrheal illness is poorly characterized, but is acute and self-limiting.

8. Target Population

All individuals are susceptible. No age or race susceptibilities have been found.

9. Analysis of Foods

Suspect food is examined microbiologically by selective enumeration techniques which can take up to 7 days. Group specificities are determined by Lancefield group-specific antisera.

10. Selected Outbreaks

Group A: Outbreaks of septic sore throat and scarlet fever were numerous before the advent of milk pasteurization. Salad bars have been suggested as possible sources of infection. Most current outbreaks have involved complex foods (i.e., salads) which were infected by a food handler with septic sore throat. One ill food handler may subsequently infect hundreds of individuals.

Group D: Outbreaks are not common and are usually the result of preparing, storing, or handling food in an unsanitary manner.

For more information on recent outbreaks see the *Morbidity and Mortality Weekly Reports* from CDC.

Giardia lamblia

1. Name of the Organism

Giardia lamblia

Giardia lamblia (intestinalis) is a single celled animal, i.e., a protozoa, that moves with the aid of five flagella. In Europe, it is sometimes referred to as *Lamblia intestinalis.*

2. Disease Name

Giardiasis is the most frequent cause of non-bacterial diarrhea in North America.

3. Nature of the Disease

Organisms that appear identical to those that cause human illness have been isolated from domestic animals (dogs and cats) and wild animals (beavers and bears). A related but morphologically distinct organism infects rodents, although rodents may be infected with human isolates in the laboratory. Human giardiasis may involve diarrhea within 1 week of ingestion of the cyst, which is the environmental survival form and infective stage of the organism. Normally illness lasts for 1 to 2 weeks, but there are cases of chronic infections lasting months to years. Chronic cases, both those with defined immune deficiencies and those without, are difficult to treat. The disease mechanism is unknown, with some investigators reporting that the organism produces a toxin while others are unable to confirm its existence. The organism has been demonstrated inside host cells in the duodenum, but most investigators think this is such an infrequent occurrence that it is not responsible for disease symptoms. Mechanical obstruction of the absorptive surface of the intestine has been proposed as a possible pathogenic mechanism, as has a synergistic relationship with some of the intestinal flora. Giardia can be excysted, cultured and encysted in vitro; new isolates have bacterial, fungal, and viral symbionts. Classically the disease was diagnosed by demonstration of the organism in stained fecal smears. Several strains of *G. lamblia* have been isolated and described through analysis of their proteins and DNA; type of strain, however, is not consistently associated with disease severity. Different individuals show various degrees of symptoms when infected with the same strain, and the symptoms of an individual may vary during the course of the disease.

Infectious Dose—Ingestion of one or more cysts may cause disease, as contrasted to most bacterial illnesses where hundreds to thousands of organisms must be consumed to produce illness.

4. Diagnosis of Human Illness

Giardia lamblia is frequently diagnosed by visualizing the organism, either the trophozoite (active reproducing form) or the cyst (the resting stage that is resistant to adverse environmental conditions) in stained preparations or unstained wet mounts with the aid of a microscope. A commercial fluorescent antibody kit is available to stain the organism. Organisms may be concentrated by sedimentation or flotation; however, these procedures reduce the number of recognizable organisms in the sample. An enzyme linked immunosorbant assay (ELISA) that detects excretory secretory products of the organism is also available. So far, the increased sensitivity of indirect serological detection has not been consistently demonstrated.

5. Associated Foods

Giardiasis is most frequently associated with the consumption of contaminated water. Five outbreaks have been traced to food contamination by infected or infested food handlers, and the possibility of infections from contaminated vegetables that are eaten raw cannot be excluded. Cool moist conditions favor the survival of the organism.

6. Relative Frequency of Disease

Giardiasis is more prevalent in children than in adults, possibly because many individuals seem to have a lasting immunity after infection. This organism is implicated in 25% of the cases of gastrointestinal disease and may be present asymptomatically. The overall incidence of infection in the United States is estimated at 2% of the population. This disease afflicts many homosexual men, both HIV-positive and HIV-negative individuals. This is presumed to be due to sexual transmission. The disease is also common in child day care centers, especially those in which diapering is done.

7. Complications About 40% of those who are diagnosed with giardiasis demonstrate disaccharide intolerance during detectable infection and up to 6 months after the infection can no longer be detected. Lactose (i.e., milk sugar) intolerance is most frequently observed. Some individuals (less than 4%) remain symptomatic more than 2 weeks; chronic infections lead to a malabsorption syndrome and severe weight loss. Chronic cases of giardiasis in immunodeficient and normal individuals are frequently refractile to drug treatment. Flagyl is normally quite effective in terminating infections. In some immune deficient individuals, giardiasis may contribute to a shortening of the life span.

8. Target Populations Giardiasis occurs throughout the population, although the prevalence is higher in children than adults. Chronic symptomatic giardiasis is more common in adults than children.

9. Food Analysis Food is analyzed by thorough surface cleaning of the suspected food and sedimentation of the organisms from the cleaning water. Feeding to specific pathogen-free animals has been used to detect the organism in large outbreaks associated with municipal water systems. The precise sensitivity of these methods has not been determined, so that negative results are questionable. Seven days may be required to detect an experimental infection.

10. Selected Outbreaks Major outbreaks are associated with contaminated water systems that do not use sand filtration or have a defect in the filtration system. The largest reported foodborne outbreak involved 24 of 36 persons who consumed macaroni salad at a picnic.

For more information on recent outbreaks see the *Morbidity and Mortality Weekly Reports* from CDC.

11. FDA Regulations or Activity

FDA is actively developing and improving methods of recovering parasitic protozoa and helminth eggs from foods. Current recovery methods are published in the FDA's Bacteriological Analytical Manual.

Cryptosporidium parvum

1. Name of the Organism

Cryptosporidium parvum

2. Disease Name

Intestinal, tracheal, or pulmonary cryptosporidiosis.

3. Nature of Acute Disease

Intestinal cryptosporidiosis is characterized by severe watery diarrhea but may, alternatively, be asymptomatic. Pulmonary and tracheal cryptosporidiosis in humans is associated with coughing and frequently a low-grade fever; these symptoms are often accompanied by severe intestinal distress.

Infectious dose—Less than 10 organisms and, presumably, one organism can initiate an infection. The mechanism of disease is not known; however, the intracellular stages of the parasite can cause severe tissue alteration.

4. Diagnosis of Human Illness

Oocysts are shed in the infected individual's feces. Sugar flotation is used to concentrate the organisms and acid fast staining is used to identify them. A commercial kit is available that uses fluorescent antibody to stain the organisms isolated from feces. Diagnosis has also been made by staining the trophozoites in intestinal and biopsy specimens. Pulmonary and tracheal cryptosporidiosis are diagnosed by biopsy and staining.

5. Food Occurrence

Cryptosporidium sp. could occur, theoretically, on any food touched by a contaminated food handler. Incidence is higher in child day care centers that serve food. Fertilizing salad vegetables with manure is another possible source of human infection. Large outbreaks are associated with contaminated water supplies.

6. Relative Frequency of the Disease

Direct human surveys indicate a prevalence of about 2% of the population in North America. Serological surveys indicate that 80% of the population has had cryptosporidiosis. The extent of illness associated with reactive sera is not known.

7. Usual Course of the Disease and Complications   Intestinal cryptosporidiosis is self-limiting in most healthy individuals, with watery diarrhea lasting 2–4 days. In some outbreaks at day care centers, diarrhea has lasted 1 to 4 weeks. To date, there is no known effective drug for the treatment of cryptosporidiosis. Immunodeficient individuals, especially AIDS patients, may have the disease for life, with the severe watery diarrhea contributing to death. Invasion of the pulmonary system may also be fatal.

8. Target Populations   In animals, the young show the most severe symptoms. For the most part, pulmonary infections are confined to those who are immunodeficient. However, an infant with a presumably normal immune system had tracheal cryptosporidiosis (although a concurrent viremia may have accounted for lowered resistance). Child day care centers, with a large susceptible population, frequently report outbreaks.

9. Analysis of Foods   The 7th edition of FDA's Bacteriological Analytical Manual will contain a method for the examination of vegetables for *Cryptosporidium* sp.

10. Selected Outbreaks   Since 1984, cryptosporidiosis has been associated with outbreaks of diarrheal illness in child day care centers throughout the United States and Canada. During 1987 a waterborne outbreak in Georgia produced illness in an estimated 13,000 individuals, and exposure to contaminated drinking water was the major distinction between those that were ill and those that were not. This was the first report of disease transmission by a municipal water system that was in compliance with all state and federal standards.

An outbreak of cryptosporidiosis associated with the consumption of apple cider is reported in MMWR 46(1):1997 Jan 10.

MMWR 45(36):1996 Sep 13 reports on an outbreak of cryptosporidiosis associated with the consumption of home-made chicken salad in Minnesota.

A non-food outbreak of cryptosporidiosis in a day-camp is reported in MMWR 45(21):1995 May 31. This report is linked to this chapter to provide reference information.

MMWR 39(20):1990 May 25 reports on a non-food related outbreak of cryptosporidiosis, but contains useful information on *Cryptosporidium* sp.

For more information on recent outbreaks see the *Morbidity and Mortality Weekly Reports* from CDC.

11. FDA Regulations or Activity

FDA is developing and improving methods for the recovery of cysts of parasitic protozoa from fresh vegetables. Current recovery methods are published in the Bacteriological Analytical Manual.

12. Education

The CDC has information on *Cryptosporidium.*

13. Other Resources

From GenBank there is a Loci index for genome *Cryptosporidium parvum.*

Hepatitis A Virus

1. Name of the Organism

Hepatitis A virus

Hepatitis A virus (HAV) is classified with the enterovirus group of the Picornaviridae family. HAV has a single molecule of RNA surrounded by a small (27 nm diameter) protein capsid and a buoyant density in CsCl of 1.33 g/ml. Many other picornaviruses cause human disease, including polioviruses, coxsackieviruses, echoviruses, and rhinoviruses (cold viruses).

2. Name of Acute Disease

The term hepatitis A (HA) or type A viral hepatitis has replaced all previous designations: infectious hepatitis, epidemic hepatitis, epidemic jaundice, catarrhal jaundice, infectious icterus, Botkins disease, and MS-1 hepatitis.

3. Nature of Disease

Hepatitis A is usually a mild illness characterized by sudden onset of fever, malaise, nausea, anorexia, and abdominal discomfort, followed in several days by jaundice. The infectious dose is unknown but presumably is 10–100 virus particles.

4. Diagnosis of Human Illness

Hepatitis A is diagnosed by finding IgM-class anti-HAV in serum collected during the acute or early convalescent phase of disease. Commercial kits are available.

5. Associated Foods

HAV is excreted in feces of infected people and can produce clinical disease when susceptible individuals consume contaminated water or foods. Cold cuts and sandwiches, fruits and fruit juices, milk and milk products, vegetables, salads, shellfish, and iced drinks are commonly implicated in outbreaks. Water, shellfish, and salads are the most frequent sources. Contamination of foods by infected workers in food processing plants and restaurants is common.

6. Frequency of Disease

Hepatitis A has a worldwide distribution occurring in both epidemic and sporadic fashions. About 22,700 cases of hepatitis A representing 38% of all hepatitis cases (5-year average from all routes of transmission) are reported annually in the U.S. In 1988 an estimated 7.3% cases were foodborne or waterborne. HAV is primarily transmitted by person-to-person contact through fecal contamination, but common-source epidemics from contaminated food and water also occur. Poor sanitation and crowding facilitate transmission. Outbreaks of HA are common in institutions, crowded house projects, and prisons and in military forces in adverse situations. In developing countries, the incidence of disease in adults is relatively low because of exposure to the virus in childhood. Most individuals 18 and older demonstrate an immunity that provides lifelong protection against reinfection. In the U.S., the percentage of adults with immunity increases with age (10% for those 18–19 years of age to 65% for those over 50). The increased number of susceptible individuals allows common source epidemics to evolve rapidly.

7. Usual Course of Disease

The incubation period for hepatitis A, which varies from 10 to 50 days (mean 30 days), is dependent upon the number of infectious particles consumed. Infection with very few particles results in longer incubation periods. The period of communicability extends from early in the incubation period to about a week after the development of jaundice. The greatest danger of spreading the disease to others occurs during the middle of the incubation period, well before the first presentation of symptoms. Many infections with HAV do not result in clinical disease, especially in children. When disease does occur, it is usually mild and recovery is complete in 1–2 weeks. Occasionally, the symptoms are severe and convalescence can take several months. Patients suffer from feeling chronically tired during convalescence, and their inability to work can cause financial loss. Less than 0.4% of the reported cases in the U.S. are fatal. These rare deaths usually occur in the elderly.

8. Target Population

All people who ingest the virus and are immunologically unprotected are susceptible to infection. Disease, however, is more common in adults than in children.

9. Analysis of Foods

The virus has not been isolated from any food associated with an outbreak. Because of the long incubation period, the suspected food is often no longer available for analysis. No satisfactory method is presently available for routine analysis of food, but sensitive molecular methods used to detect HAV in water and clinical specimens should prove useful to detect virus in foods. Among those, the PCR amplification method seems particularly promising.

10. Selected Outbreaks

Hepatitis A is endemic throughout much of the world. Major national epidemics occurred in 1954, 1961 and 1971. Although no major epidemic occurred in the 1980s, the incidence of hepatitis A in the U.S. increased 58% from 1983 to 1989. Foods have been implicated in over 30 outbreaks since 1983. The most recent ones and the suspected contaminated foods include:

- 1987—Louisville, Kentucky. Suspected source: imported lettuce.
- 1988—Alaska. Ice-slush beverage prepared in a local market.—North Carolina. Iced tea prepared in a restaurant.—Florida. Raw oysters harvested from nonapproved bed.
- 1989—Washington. Unidentified food in a restaurant chain.
- 1990—North Georgia. Frozen strawberries.— Montana. Frozen strawberries.—Baltimore. Shellfish.

A summary of foodborne Hepatitis A outbreaks in Missouri, Wisconsin, and Alaska is found in MMWR 42(27):1993 Jul 16.

MMWR 39(14):1990 Apr 13 summarizes foodborne outbreaks of Hepatitis A in Alaska, Florida, North Carolina, Washington.

For more information on recent outbreaks see the
Morbidity and Mortality Weekly Reports from CDC.

Rotavirus

1. Name of the Organism

Rotavirus
   Rotaviruses are classified with the Reoviridae family. They have a genome consisting of 11 double-stranded RNA segments surrounded by a distinctive two-layered protein capsid. Particles are 70 nm in diameter and have a buoyant density of 1.36 g/ml in CsCl. Six serological groups have been identified, three of which (groups A, B, and C) infect humans.

2. Name of Acute Disease

Rotaviruses cause acute gastroenteritis. Infantile diarrhea, winter diarrhea, acute nonbacterial infectious gastroenteritis, and acute viral gastroenteritis are names applied to the infection caused by the most common and widespread group A rotavirus.

3. Nature of Disease

Rotavirus gastroenteritis is a self-limiting, mild to severe disease characterized by vomiting, watery diarrhea, and low-grade fever. The infective dose is presumed to be 10–100 infectious viral particles. Because a person with rotavirus diarrhea often excretes large numbers of virus (10^8–10^{10} infectious particles/ml of feces), infection doses can be readily acquired through contaminated hands, objects, or utensils. Asymptomatic rotavirus excretion has been well documented and may play a role in perpetuating endemic disease.

4. Diagnosis of Human Illness

Specific diagnosis of the disease is made by identification of the virus in the patient's stool. Enzyme immunoassay (EIA) is the test most widely used to screen clinical specimens, and several commercial kits are available for group A rotavirus. Electron microscopy (EM) and polyacrylamide gel electrophoresis (PAGE) are used in some laboratories in addition or as an alternative to EIA. A reverse transcription-polymerase chain reaction (RT-PCR) has been developed to detect and identify all three groups of human rotaviruses.

5. Associated Foods

Rotaviruses are transmitted by the fecal-oral route. Person-to-person spread through contaminated hands is probably the most important means by which rotaviruses are transmitted in close communities such as pediatric and geriatric wards, day care centers and family homes. Infected food handlers may contaminate foods that require handling and no further cooking, such as salads, fruits, and hors d'oeuvres. Rotaviruses are quite stable in the environment and have been found in estuary samples at levels as high as 1–5 infectious particles/gal. Sanitary measures adequate for bacteria and parasites seem to be ineffective in endemic control of rotavirus, as similar incidence of rotavirus infection is observed in countries with both high and low health standards.

6. Frequency of Disease

Group A rotavirus is endemic worldwide. It is the leading cause of severe diarrhea among infants and children, and accounts for about half of the cases requiring hospitalization. Over 3 million cases of rotavirus gastroenteritis occur annually in the U.S. In temperate areas, it occurs primarily in the winter, but in the tropics it occurs throughout the year. The number attributable to food contamination is unknown.

Group B rotavirus, also called adult diarrhea rotavirus or ADRV, has caused major epidemics of severe diarrhea affecting thousands of persons of all ages in China.

Group C rotavirus has been associated with rare and sporadic cases of diarrhea in children in many countries. However, the first outbreaks were reported from Japan and England.

7. Usual Course of Disease

The incubation period ranges from 1–3 days. Symptoms often start with vomiting followed by 4–8 days of diarrhea. Temporary lactose intolerance may occur. Recovery is usually complete. However, severe diarrhea without fluid and electrolyte replacement may result in death. Childhood mortality caused by rotavirus is relatively low in the U.S., with an estimated 100 cases/year, but reaches almost 1 million cases/year worldwide. Association with other enteric pathogens may play a role in the severity of the disease.

8. Target Populations

Humans of all ages are susceptible to rotavirus infection. Children 6 months to 2 years of age, premature infants, the elderly, and the immunocompromised are particularly prone to more severe symptoms caused by infection with group A rotavirus.

9. Analysis of Foods

The virus has not been isolated from any food associated with an outbreak, and no satisfactory method is available for routine analysis of food. However, it should be possible to apply procedures that have been used to detect the virus in water and in clinical specimens, such as enzyme immunoassays, gene probing, and PCR amplification to food analysis.

10. Selected Outbreaks

Outbreaks of group A rotavirus diarrhea are common among hospitalized infants, young children attending day care centers, and elderly persons in nursing homes. Among adults, multiple foods served in banquets were implicated in 2 outbreaks. An outbreak due to contaminated municipal water occurred in Colorado, 1981.

Several large outbreaks of group B rotavirus involving millions of persons as a result of sewage contamination of drinking water supplies have occurred in China since 1982. Although to date outbreaks caused by group B rotavirus have been confined to mainland China, seroepidemiological surveys have indicated lack of immunity to this group of virus in the U.S.

The newly recognized group C rotavirus has been implicated in rare and isolated cases of gastroenteritis. However, it was associated with three outbreaks among school children: one in Japan, 1989, and two in England, 1990.

For a discussion of rotavirus surveillance in the US, see MMWR 40(5):1991 Feb 8.

For more information on recent outbreaks see the *Morbidity and Mortality Weekly Reports* from CDC.

11. Other Resources

From GenBank there is a Loci index for genome Rotavirus sp.

The Norwalk Virus Family

1. Name of the Organism

The Norwalk virus family

Norwalk virus is the prototype of a family of unclassified small round structured viruses (SRSVs) which may be related to the caliciviruses. They contain a positive strand RNA genome of 7.5 kb and a single structural protein of about 60 kDa. The 27–32 nm viral particles have a buoyant density of 1.39–1.40 g/ml in CsCl. The family consists of several serologically distinct groups of viruses that have been named after the places where the outbreaks occurred. In the U.S., the Norwalk and Montgomery County agents are serologically related but distinct from the Hawaii and Snow Mountain agents. The Taunton, Moorcroft, Barnett, and Amulree agents were identified in the U.K., and the Sapporo and Otofuke agents in Japan. Their serological relationships remain to be determined.

2. Name of Acute Disease

Common names of the illness caused by the Norwalk and Norwalk-like viruses are viral gastroenteritis, acute nonbacterial gastroenteritis, food poisoning, and food infection.

3. Nature of Disease

The disease is self-limiting, mild, and characterized by nausea, vomiting, diarrhea, and abdominal pain. Headache and low-grade fever may occur. The infectious dose is unknown but presumed to be low.

4. Diagnosis of Human Illness

Specific diagnosis of the disease can only be made by a few laboratories possessing reagents from human volunteer studies. Identification of the virus can be made on early stool specimens using immune electron microscopy and various immunoassays. Confirmation often requires demonstration of seroconversion, the presence of specific IgM antibody, or a four-fold rise in antibody titer to Norwalk virus on paired acute-convalescent sera.

5. Associated Foods

Norwalk gastroenteritis is transmitted by the fecal-oral route via contaminated water and foods. Secondary person-to-person transmission has been documented. Water is the most common source of outbreaks and may include water from municipal supplies, well, recreational lakes, swimming pools, and water stored aboard cruise ships.

Shellfish and salad ingredients are the foods most often implicated in Norwalk outbreaks. Ingestion of raw or insufficiently steamed clams and oysters poses a high risk for infection with Norwalk virus. Foods other than shellfish are contaminated by ill food handlers.

6. Frequency of Disease

Only the common cold is reported more frequently than viral gastroenteritis as a cause of illness in the U.S. Although viral gastroenteritis is caused by a number of viruses, it is estimated that Norwalk viruses are responsible for about 1/3 of the cases not involving the 6-to-24-month age group. In developing countries the percentage of individuals who have developed immunity is very high at an early age. In the U.S. the percentage increases gradually with age, reaching 50% in the population over 18 years of age. Immunity, however, is not permanent and reinfection can occur.

7. Usual Course of Disease and Some Complications

A mild and brief illness usually develops 24–48 hours after contaminated food or water is consumed and lasts for 24–60 hours. Severe illness or hospitalization is very rare.

8. Target Populations

All individuals who ingest the virus and who have not (within 24 months) had an infection with the same or related strain, are susceptible to infection and can develop the symptoms of gastroenteritis. Disease is more frequent in adults and older children than in the very young.

9. Analysis of Foods

The virus has been identified in clams and oysters by radioimmunoassay. The genome of Norwalk virus has been cloned and development of gene probes and PCR amplification techniques to detect the virus in clinical specimens and possibly in food are under way.

10. Selected Outbreaks

Foodborne outbreaks of gastroenteritis caused by Norwalk virus are often related to consumption of raw shellfish. Frequent and widespread outbreaks, reaching epidemic proportions, occurred in Australia (1978) and in the state of New York (1982) among consumers of raw clams and oysters. From 1983 to 1987, ten well documented outbreaks caused by Norwalk virus were reported in the U.S., involving a variety of foods: fruits, salads, eggs, clams, and bakery items.

Preliminary evidence suggests that large outbreaks of gastroenteritis which occurred in Pennsylvania and Delaware in September, 1987, were caused by Norwalk virus. The source of both outbreaks was traced to ice made with water from a contaminated well. In Pennsylvania, the ice was consumed at a football game, and in Delaware, at a cocktail party. Norwalk virus is also suspected to have caused an outbreak aboard a cruise ship in Hawaii in 1990. Fresh fruits were the probable vehicle of contamination.

Snow Mountain virus was implicated in an outbreak in a retirement community in California (1988) which resulted in two deaths. Illness was associated with consumption of shrimp probably contaminated by food handlers.

For outbreaks of Norwalk virus see MMWR 42(49):1993 Dec 17 and this MMWR 43(24):1994 Jun 24 as well.

The multistate outbreak of viral gastroenteritis associated with consumption of oysters from Apalachicola Bay, Florida, December 1994-January 1995 is reported in MMWR 44(2):1995 Jan 20.

For more information on recent outbreaks see the *Morbidity and Mortality Weekly Reports* from CDC.

Other Gastroenteritis Viruses

1. Name of the Organism

Other viruses associated with gastroenteritis

Although the rotavirus and the Norwalk family of viruses are the leading causes of viral gastroenteritis, a number of other viruses have been implicated in outbreaks, including astroviruses, caliciviruses, enteric adenoviruses and parvovirus. Astroviruses, caliciviruses, and the Norwalk family of viruses possess well-defined surface structures and are sometimes identified as "small round structured viruses" or SRSVs. Viruses with smooth edge and no discernible surface structure are designated "featureless viruses" or "small round viruses" (SRVs). These agents resemble enterovirus or parvovirus, and may be related to them.

Astroviruses are unclassified viruses which contain a single positive strand of RNA of about 7.5 kb surrounded by a protein capsid of 28–30 nm diameter. A five or six pointed star shape can be observed on the particles under the electron microscope. Mature virions contain two major coat proteins of about 33 kDa each and have a buoyant density in CsCl of 1.38–1.40 g/ml. At least five human serotypes have been identified in England. The Marin County agent found in the U.S. is serologically related to astrovirus type 5.

Caliciviruses are classified in the family Caliciviridae. They contain a single strand of RNA surrounded by a protein capsid of 31–40 nm diameter. Mature virions have cup-shaped indentations which give them a "Star of David" appearance in the electron microscope. The particle contains a single major coat protein of 60 kDa and have a buoyant density in CsCl of 1.36–1.39 g/ml. Four serotypes have been identified in England.

Enteric adenoviruses represent serotypes 40 and 41 of the family Adenoviridae. These viruses contain a double-stranded DNA surrounded by a distinctive protein capsid of about 70 nm diameter. Mature virions have a buoyant density in CsCl of about 1.345 g/ml.

Parvoviruses belong to the family Parvoviridae, the only group of animal viruses to contain linear single-stranded DNA. The DNA genome is surrounded by a protein capsid of about 22 nm diameter. The buoyant density of the particle in CsCl is 1.39–1.42 g/ml. The Ditchling, Wollan, Paramatta, and cockle agents are candidate parvoviruses associated with human gastroenteritis.

2. Name of Acute Disease

Common names of the illness caused by these viruses are acute nonbacterial infectious gastroenteritis and viral gastroenteritis.

3. Nature of Disease

Viral gastroenteritis is usually a mild illness characterized by nausea, vomiting, diarrhea, malaise, abdominal pain, headache, and fever. The infectious dose is not known but is presumed to be low.

4. Diagnosis of Human Illness

Specific diagnosis of the disease can be made by some laboratories possessing appropriate reagents. Identification of the virus present in early acute stool samples is made by immune electron microscopy and various enzyme immunoassays. Confirmation often requires demonstration of seroconversion to the agent by serological tests on acute and convalescent serum pairs.

5. Associated Foods

Viral gastroenteritis is transmitted by the fecal-oral route via person-to-person contact or ingestion of contaminated foods and water. Ill food handlers may contaminate foods that are not further cooked before consumption. Enteric adenovirus may also be transmitted by the respiratory route. Shellfish have been implicated in illness caused by a parvo-like virus.

6. Frequency of Disease

Astroviruses cause sporadic gastroenteritis in children under 4 years of age and account for about 4% of the cases hospitalized for diarrhea. Most American and British children over 10 years of age have antibodies to the virus.

Caliciviruses infect children between 6 and 24 months of age and account for about 3% of hospital admissions for diarrhea. By 6 years of age, more than 90% of all children have developed immunity to the illness.

The enteric adenovirus causes 5–20% of the gastroenteritis in young children, and is the second most common cause of gastroenteritis in this age group. By 4 years of age, 85% of all children have developed immunity to the disease. Parvo-like viruses have been implicated in a number of shellfish-associated outbreaks, but the frequency of disease is unknown.

7. Usual Course of Disease and Some Complications

A mild, self-limiting illness usually develops 10 to 70 hours after contaminated food or water is consumed and lasts for 2 to 9 days. The clinical features are milder but otherwise indistinguishable from rotavirus gastroenteritis. Co-infections with other enteric agents may result in more severe illness lasting a longer period of time.

8. Target Population

The target populations for astro- and caliciviruses are young children and the elderly. Only young children seem to develop illness caused by the enteric adenoviruses. Infection with these viruses is widespread and seems to result in development of immunity. Parvoviruses infect all age groups and probably do not illicit a permanent immunity.

9. Analysis of Foods

Only a parvovirus-like agent (cockle) has been isolated from seafood associated with an outbreak. Although foods are not routinely analyzed for these viruses, it may be possible to apply current immunological procedures to detect viruses in clinical specimens. Gene probes and PCR detection methods are currently being developed.

10. Selected Outbreaks

Outbreaks of astrovirus and calicivirus occur mainly in child care settings and nursing homes. In the past decade, 7 outbreaks of calicivirus and 4 of astrovirus have been reported from England and Japan. In California, an outbreak caused by an astrovirus, the Marin County agent, occurred among elderly patients in a convalescent hospital. No typical calicivirus has been implicated in outbreaks in the U.S. However, if Norwalk and Norwalk-like viruses prove to be caliciviruses, they would account for most food and waterborne outbreaks of gastroenteritis in this country.

Outbreaks of adenovirus have been reported in England and Japan, all involving children in hospitals or day care centers.

The small, featureless, parvo-like viruses caused outbreaks of gastroenteritis in primary and secondary schools in England (Ditchling and Wollan) and Australia (Paramatta). The cockle agent caused a large community-wide outbreak in England (1977) associated with consumption of contaminated seafood. Parvo-like viruses were also implicated in several outbreaks which occurred in the States of New York and Louisiana in 1982–1983.

For more information on recent outbreaks see the *Morbidity and Mortality Weekly Reports* from CDC.

Various Shellfish-Associated Toxins

1. Name of Toxins

Various Shellfish-Associated

Shellfish poisoning is caused by a group of toxins elaborated by planktonic algae (dinoflagellates, in most cases) upon which the shellfish feed. The toxins are accumulated and sometimes metabolized by the shellfish. The 20 toxins responsible for paralytic shellfish poisonings (PSP) are all derivatives of saxitoxin. Diarrheic shellfish poisoning (DSP) is presumably caused by a group of high molecular weight polyethers, including okadaic acid, the dinophysis toxins, the pectenotoxins, and yessotoxin. Neurotoxic shellfish poisoning (NSP) is the result of exposure to a group of polyethers called brevetoxins. Amnesic shellfish poisoning (ASP) is caused by the unusual amino acid, domoic acid, as the contaminant of shellfish.

2. Name of the Acute Diseases

Shellfish Poisoning: Paralytic Shellfish Poisoning (PSP), Diarrheic Shellfish Poisoning (DSP), Neurotoxic Shellfish Poisoning (NSP), Amnesic Shellfish Poisoning (ASP).

3. Nature of the Diseases

Ingestion of contaminated shellfish results in a wide variety of symptoms, depending upon the toxin(s) present, their concentrations in the shellfish and the amount of contaminated shellfish consumed. In the case of PSP, the effects are predominantly neurological and include tingling, burning, numbness, drowsiness, incoherent speech, and respiratory paralysis. Less well characterized are the symptoms associated with DSP, NSP, and ASP. DSP is primarily observed as a generally mild gastrointestinal disorder, i.e., nausea, vomiting, diarrhea, and abdominal pain accompanied by chills, headache, and fever. Both gastrointestinal and neurological symptoms characterize NSP, including tingling and numbness of lips, tongue, and throat, muscular aches, dizziness, reversal of the sensations of hot and cold, diarrhea, and vomiting. ASP is characterized by gastrointestinal disorders (vomiting, diarrhea, abdominal pain) and neurological problems (confusion, memory loss, disorientation, seizure, coma).

4. Normal Course of the Disease

PSP: Symptoms of the disease develop fairly rapidly, within 0.5 to 2 hours after ingestion of the shellfish, depending on the amount of toxin consumed. In severe cases respiratory paralysis is common, and death may occur if respiratory support is not provided. When such support is applied within 12 hours of exposure, recovery usually is complete, with no lasting side effects. In unusual cases, because of the weak hypotensive action of the toxin, death may occur from cardiovascular collapse despite respiratory support.

NSP: Onset of this disease occurs within a few minutes to a few hours; duration is fairly short, from a few hours to several days. Recovery is complete with few after effects; no fatalities have been reported.

DSP: Onset of the disease, depending on the dose of toxin ingested, may be as little as 30 minutes to 2 to 3 hours, with symptoms of the illness lasting as long as 2 to 3 days. Recovery is complete with no after effects; the disease is generally not life threatening.

ASP: The toxicosis is characterized by the onset of gastrointestinal symptoms within 24 hours; neurological symptoms occur within 48 hours. The toxicosis is particularly serious in elderly patients, and includes symptoms reminiscent of Alzheimer's disease. All fatalities to date have involved elderly patients.

5. Diagnosis of Human Illnesses

Diagnosis of shellfish poisoning is based entirely on observed symptomatology and recent dietary history.

6. Associated Foods

All shellfish (filter-feeding molluscs) are potentially toxic. However, PSP is generally associated with mussels, clams, cockles, and scallops; NSP with shellfish harvested along the Florida coast and the Gulf of Mexico; DSP with mussels, oysters, and scallops, and ASP with mussels.

7. Relative Frequency of Disease

Good statistical data on the occurrence and severity of shellfish poisoning are largely unavailable, which undoubtedly reflects the inability to measure the true incidence of the disease. Cases are frequently misdiagnosed and, in general, infrequently reported. Of these toxicoses, the most serious from a public health perspective appears to be PSP. The extreme potency of the PSP toxins has, in the past, resulted in an unusually high mortality rate.

8. Target Populations

All humans are susceptible to shellfish poisoning. Elderly people are apparently predisposed to the severe neurological effects of the ASP toxin. A disproportionate number of PSP cases occur among tourists or others who are not native to the location where the toxic shellfish are harvested. This may be due to disregard for either official quarantines or traditions of safe consumption, both of which tend to protect the local population.

9. Analysis of Foods

The mouse bioassay has historically been the most universally applied technique for examining shellfish (especially for PSP); other bioassay procedures have been developed but not generally applied. Unfortunately, the dose-survival times for the DSP toxins in the mouse assay fluctuate considerably and fatty acids interfere with the assay, giving false-positive results; consequently, a suckling mouse assay that has been developed and used for control of DSP measures fluid accumulation after injection of the shellfish extract. In recent years considerable effort has been applied to development of chemical assays to replace these bioassays. As a result a good high performance liquid chromatography (HPLC) procedure has been developed to identify individual PSP toxins (detection limit for saxitoxin = 20 fg/100 g of meats; 0.2 ppm), an excellent HPLC procedure (detection limit for okadaic acid = 400 ng/g; 0.4 ppm), a commercially available immunoassay (detection limit for okadaic acid = 1 fg/100 g of meats; 0.01 ppm) for DSP and a totally satisfactory HPLC procedure for ASP (detection limit for domoic acid = 750 ng/g; 0.75 ppm).

10. Selected Outbreaks

PSP is associated with relatively few outbreaks, most likely because of the strong control programs in the United States that prevent human exposure to toxic shellfish. That PSP can be a serious public health problem, however, was demonstrated in Guatemala, where an outbreak of 187 cases with 26 deaths, recorded in 1987, resulted from ingestion of a clam soup. The outbreak led to the establishment of a control program over shellfish harvested in Guatemala.

ASP first came to the attention of public health authorities in 1987 when 156 cases of acute intoxication occurred as a result of ingestion of cultured blue mussels *(Mytilus edulis)* harvested off Prince Edward Island, in eastern Canada; 22 individuals were hospitalized and three elderly patients eventually died.

The occurrence of DSP in Europe is sporadic, continuous and presumably widespread (anecdotal). DSP poisoning has not been confirmed in U.S. seafood, but the organisms that produce DSP are present in U.S. waters. An outbreak of DSP was recently confirmed in Eastern Canada. Outbreaks of NSP are sporadic and continuous along the Gulf coast of Florida and were recently reported in North Carolina and Texas.

For more information on recent outbreaks see the *Morbidity and Mortality Weekly Reports* from CDC.

Scombrotoxin

1. Name of Toxin

Scombrotoxin

2. Name of Acute Disease   Scombroid Poisoning (also called Histamine Poisoning)

Scombroid poisoning is caused by the ingestion of foods that contain high levels of histamine and possibly other vasoactive amines and compounds. Histamine and other amines are formed by the growth of certain bacteria and the subsequent action of their decarboxylase enzymes on histidine and other amino acids in food, either during the production of a product such as Swiss cheese or by spoilage of foods such as fishery products, particularly tuna or mahi mahi. However, any food that contains the appropriate amino acids and is subjected to certain bacterial contamination and growth may lead to scombroid poisoning when ingested.

3. Nature of Disease   Initial symptoms may include a tingling or burning sensation in the mouth, a rash on the upper body and a drop in blood pressure. Frequently, headaches and itching of the skin are encountered. The symptoms may progress to nausea, vomiting, and diarrhea and may require hospitalization, particularly in the case of elderly or impaired patients.

4. Normal Course of Disease   The onset of intoxication symptoms is rapid, ranging from immediate to 30 minutes. The duration of the illness is usually 3 hours, but may last several days.

5. Diagnosis of Human Illness   Diagnosis of the illness is usually based on the patient's symptoms, time of onset, and the effect of treatment with antihistamine medication. The suspected food must be analyzed within a few hours for elevated levels of histamine to confirm a diagnosis.

6. Associated Foods   Fishery products that have been implicated in scombroid poisoning include the tunas (e.g., skipjack and yellowfin), mahi mahi, bluefish, sardines, mackerel, amberjack, and abalone. Many other products also have caused the toxic effects. The primary cheese involved in intoxications has been Swiss cheese. The toxin forms in a food when certain bacteria are present and time and temperature permit their growth. Distribution of the toxin within an individual fish fillet or between cans in a case lot can be uneven, with some sections of a product causing illnesses and others not. Neither cooking, canning, nor freezing reduces the toxic effect. Common sensory examination by the consumer cannot ensure the absence or presence of the toxin. Chemical testing is the only reliable test for evaluation of a product.

7. Relative Frequency of Disease

Scombroid poisoning remains one of the most common forms of fish poisoning in the United States. Even so, incidents of poisoning often go unreported because of the lack of required reporting, a lack of information by some medical personnel, and confusion with the symptoms of other illnesses. Difficulties with underreporting are a worldwide problem. In the United States from 1968 to 1980, 103 incidents of intoxication involving 827 people were reported. For the same period in Japan, where the quality of fish is a national priority, 42 incidents involving 4,122 people were recorded. Since 1978, 2 actions by FDA have reduced the frequency of intoxications caused by specific products. A defect action level for histamine in canned tuna resulted in increased industry quality control. Secondly, block-listing of mahi mahi reduced the level of fish imported to the United States.

8. Target Population

All humans are susceptible to scombroid poisoning; however, the symptoms can be severe for the elderly and for those taking medications such as isoniazid. Because of the worldwide network for harvesting, processing, and distributing fishery products, the impact of the problem is not limited to specific geographical areas of the United States or consumption pattern. These foods are sold for use in homes, schools, hospitals, and restaurants as fresh, frozen, or processed products.

9. Analysis of Foods

An official method was developed at FDA to determine histamine, using a simple alcoholic extraction and quantitation by fluorescence spectroscopy. There are other untested procedures in the literature.

10. Selected Outbreaks

Several large outbreaks of scombroid poisoning have been reported. In 1970, some 40 children in a school lunch program became ill from imported canned tuna. In 1973, more than 200 consumers across the United States were affected by domestic canned tuna. In 1979–1980 more than 200 individuals became ill after consuming imported frozen mahi mahi. Symptoms varied with each incident. In the 1973 situation, of the interviewed patients, 86% experienced nausea, 55% diarrhea, 44% headaches and 32% rashes.

Other incidents of intoxication have resulted from the consumption of canned abalone-like products, canned anchovies, and fresh and frozen amberjack, bluefish sole, and scallops. In particular, shipments of unfrozen fish packed in refrigerated containers have posed a significant problem because of inadequate temperature control.

For more information on recent outbreaks see the *Morbidity and Mortality Weekly Reports* from CDC.

Mushroom Toxins

1. Name of Toxin(s)   Amanitin, Gyromitrin, Orellanine, Muscarine, Ibotenic Acid, Muscimol, Psilocybin, Coprine

2. Name of Acute Disease   Mushroom Poisoning, Toadstool Poisoning

Mushroom poisoning is caused by the consumption of raw or cooked fruiting bodies (mushrooms, toadstools) of a number of species of higher fungi. The term toadstool (from the German Todesstuhl, death's stool) is commonly given to poisonous mushrooms, but for individuals who are not experts in mushroom identification there are generally no easily recognizable differences between poisonous and nonpoisonous species. Old wives' tales notwithstanding, there is no general rule of thumb for distinguishing edible mushrooms and poisonous toadstools. The toxins involved in mushroom poisoning are produced naturally by the fungi themselves, and each individual specimen of a toxic species should be considered equally poisonous. Most mushrooms that cause human poisoning cannot be made nontoxic by cooking, canning, freezing, or any other means of processing. Thus, the only way to avoid poisoning is to avoid consumption of the toxic species. Poisonings in the United States occur most commonly when hunters of wild mushrooms (especially novices) misidentify and consume a toxic species, when recent immigrants collect and consume a poisonous American species that closely resembles an edible wild mushroom from their native land, or when mushrooms that contain psychoactive compounds are intentionally consumed by persons who desire these effects.

3. Nature of Disease(s)   Mushroom poisonings are generally acute and are manifested by a variety of symptoms and prognoses, depending on the amount and species consumed. Because the chemistry of many of the mushroom toxins (especially the less deadly ones) is still unknown and positive identification of the mushrooms is often difficult or impossible, mushroom poisonings are generally categorized by their physiological effects. There are four categories of mushroom toxins: protoplasmic poisons (poisons that result in generalized destruction of cells, followed by organ failure); neurotoxins (compounds that cause neurological symptoms such as profuse sweating, coma, convulsions, hallucinations, excitement, depression, spastic colon); gastrointestinal irritants (compounds that produce rapid, transient nausea, vomiting, abdominal cramping, and diarrhea); and disulfiram-like toxins. Mushrooms in this last category are generally nontoxic and produce no symptoms unless alcohol is consumed within 72 hours after eating them, in which case a short-lived acute toxic syndrome is produced.

4. Normal Course of Disease(s)   The normal course of the disease varies with the dose and the mushroom species eaten. Each poisonous species contains one or more toxic compounds which are unique to few other species. Therefore, cases of mushroom poisonings generally do not resemble each other unless they are caused by the same or very closely related mushroom species. Almost all mushroom poisonings may be grouped in one of the categories outlined above.

Protoplasmic Poisons

Amatoxins.   Several mushroom species, including the Death Cap or Destroying *Angel (Amanita phalloides, A. virosa)*, the Fool's Mushroom *(A. verna)* and several of their relatives, along with the Autumn Skullcap *(Galerina autumnalis)* and some of its relatives, produce a family of cyclic octapeptides called amanitins. Poisoning by the amanitins is characterized by a long latent period (range 6–48 hours, average 6–15 hours) during which the patient shows no symptoms. Symptoms appear at the end of the latent period in the form of sudden, severe seizures of abdominal pain, persistent vomiting and watery diarrhea, extreme thirst, and lack of urine production. If this early phase is survived, the patient may appear to recover for a short time, but this period will generally be followed by a rapid and severe loss of strength, prostration, and pain-caused restlessness. Death in 50–90% of the cases from progressive and irreversible liver, kidney, cardiac, and skeletal muscle damage may follow within 48 hours (large dose), but the disease more typically lasts 6 to 8 days in adults and 4 to 6 days in children. Two or three days after the onset of the later phase, jaundice, cyanosis, and coldness of the skin occur. Death usually follows a period of coma and occasionally convulsions. If recovery occurs, it generally requires at least a month and is accompanied by enlargement of the liver. Autopsy will usually reveal fatty degeneration and necrosis of the liver and kidney.

Hydrazines.   Certain species of False Morel (*Gyromitra esculenta* and *G. gigas*) contain the protoplasmic poison gyromitrin, a volatile hydrazine derivative. Poisoning by this toxin superficially resembles Amanita poisoning but is less severe. There is generally a latent period of 6–10 hours after ingestion during which no symptoms are evident, followed by sudden onset of abdominal discomfort (a feeling of fullness), severe headache, vomiting, and sometimes diarrhea. The toxin affects primarily the liver, but there are additional disturbances to blood cells and the central nervous system. The mortality rate is relatively low (2–4%). Poisonings with symptoms almost identical to those produced by Gyromitra have also been reported after ingestion of the Early False Morel *(Verpa bohemica).* The toxin is presumed to be related to gyromitrin but has not yet been identified.

Orellanine.   The final type of protoplasmic poisoning is caused by the Sorrel Webcap mushroom *(Cortinarius orellanus)* and some of its relatives. This mushroom produces orellanine, which causes a type of poisoning characterized by an extremely long asymptomatic latent period of 3 to 14 days. An intense, burning thirst (polydipsia) and excessive urination (polyuria) are the first symptoms. This may be followed by nausea, headache, muscular pains, chills, spasms, and loss of consciousness. In severe cases, severe renal tubular necrosis and kidney failure may result in death (15%) several weeks after the poisoning. Fatty degeneration of the liver and severe inflammatory changes in the intestine accompany the renal damage, and recovery in less severe cases may require several months.

Neurotoxins

Poisonings by mushrooms that cause neurological problems may be divided into three groups, based on the type of symptoms produced, and named for the substances responsible for these symptoms.

Muscarine Poisoning. Ingestion of any number of *Inocybe* or *Clitocybe* species (e.g., *Inocybe geophylla, Clitocybe dealbata*) results in an illness characterized primarily by profuse sweating. This effect is caused by the presence in these mushrooms of high levels (3–4%) of muscarine. Muscarine poisoning is characterized by increased salivation, perspiration, and lacrimation within 15 to 30 minutes after ingestion of the mushroom. With large doses, these symptoms may be followed by abdominal pain, severe nausea, diarrhea, blurred vision, and labored breathing. Intoxication generally subsides within 2 hours. Deaths are rare, but may result from cardiac or respiratory failure in severe cases.

Ibotenic Acid/Muscimol Poisoning. The Fly Agaric *(Amanita muscaria)* and Panthercap *(Amanita pantherina)* mushrooms both produce ibotenic acid and muscimol. Both substances produce the same effects, but muscimol is approximately 5 times more potent than ibotenic acid. Symptoms of poisoning generally occur within 1–2 hours after ingestion of the mushrooms. An initial abdominal discomfort may be present or absent, but the chief symptoms are drowsiness and dizziness (sometimes accompanied by sleep), followed by a period of hyperactivity, excitability, illusions, and delirium. Periods of drowsiness may alternate with periods of excitement, but symptoms generally fade within a few hours. Fatalities rarely occur in adults, but in children, accidental consumption of large quantities of these mushrooms may cause convulsions, coma, and other neurologic problems for up to 12 hours.

Psilocybin Poisoning. A number of mushrooms belonging to the genera *Psilocybe, Panaeolus, Copelandia, Gymnopilus, Conocybe,* and *Pluteus,* when ingested, produce a syndrome similar to alcohol intoxication (sometimes accompanied by hallucinations). Several of these mushrooms (e.g., *Psilocybe cubensis, P. mexicana, Conocybe cyanopus)* are eaten for their psychotropic effects in religious ceremonies of certain native American tribes, a practice which dates to the pre-Columbian era. The toxic effects are caused by psilocin and psilocybin. Onset of symptoms is usually rapid and the effects generally subside within 2 hours. Poisonings by these mushrooms are rarely fatal in adults and may be distinguished from ibotenic acid poisoning by the absence of drowsiness or coma. The most severe cases of psilocybin poisoning occur in small children, where large doses may cause the hallucinations accompanied by fever, convulsions, coma, and death. These mushrooms are generally small, brown, nondescript, and not particularly fleshy; they are seldom mistaken for food fungi by innocent hunters of wild mushrooms. Poisonings caused by intentional ingestion of these mushrooms by people with no legitimate religious justification must be handled with care, since the only cases likely to be seen by the physician are overdoses or intoxications caused by a combination of the mushroom and some added psychotropic substance (such as PCP).

Gastrointestinal Irritants

Numerous mushrooms, including the Green Gill (*Chlorophyllum molybdites*), Gray Pinkgill (*Entoloma lividum*), Tigertop (*Tricholoma pardinum*), Jack O'Lantern (*Omphalotus illudens*), Naked Brimcap (*Paxillus involutus*), Sickener (*Russula emetica*), Early False Morel (*Verpa bohemica*), Horse mushroom (*Agaricus arvensis*) and Pepper bolete (*Boletus piperatus*), contain toxins that can cause gastrointestinal distress, including but not limited to nausea, vomiting, diarrhea, and abdominal cramps. In many ways these symptoms are similar to those caused by the deadly protoplasmic poisons. The chief and diagnostic difference is that poisonings caused by these mushrooms have a rapid onset, rather than the delayed onset seen in protoplasmic poisonings. Some mushrooms (including the first five species mentioned above) may cause vomiting and/or diarrhea which lasts for several days. Fatalities caused by these mushrooms are relatively rare and are associated with dehydration and electrolyte imbalances caused by diarrhea and vomiting, especially in debilitated, very young, or very old patients. Replacement of fluids and other appropriate supportive therapy will prevent death in these cases. The chemistry of the toxins responsible for this type of poisoning is virtually unknown, but may be related to the presence in some mushrooms of unusual sugars, amino acids, peptides, resins, and other compounds.

Disulfiram-Like Poisoning

The Inky Cap Mushroom *(Coprinus atramentarius)* is most commonly responsible for this poisoning, although a few other species have also been implicated. A complicating factor in this type of intoxication is that this species is generally considered edible (i.e., no illness results when eaten in the absence of alcoholic beverages). The mushroom produces an unusual amino acid, coprine, which is converted to cyclopropanone hydrate in the human body. This compound interferes with the breakdown of alcohol, and consumption of alcoholic beverages within 72 hours after eating it will cause headache, nausea and vomiting, flushing, and cardiovascular disturbances that last for 2–3 hours.

Miscellaneous Poisonings

Young fruiting bodies of the sulfur shelf fungus *Laetiporus sulphureus* are considered edible. However, ingestion of this shelf fungus has caused digestive upset and other symptoms in adults and visual hallucinations and ataxia in a child.

5. Diagnosis of Human Illness A clinical testing procedure is currently available only for the most serious types of mushroom toxins, the amanitins. The commercially available method uses a 3H-radioimmunoassay (RIA) test kit and can detect sub-nanogram levels of toxin in urine and plasma. Unfortunately, it requires a 2-hour incubation period, and this is an excruciating delay in a type of poisoning which the clinician generally does not see until a day or two has passed. A 125I-based kit which overcomes this problem has recently been reported, but has not yet reached the clinic. A sensitive and rapid HPLC technique has been reported in the literature even more recently, but it has not yet seen clinical application. Since most clinical laboratories in this country do not use even the older RIA technique, diagnosis is based entirely on symptomology and recent dietary history. Despite the fact that cases of mushroom poisoning may be broken down into a relatively small number of categories based on symptomatology, positive botanical identification of the mushroom species consumed remains the only means of unequivocally determining the particular type of intoxication involved, and it is still vitally important to obtain such accurate identification as quickly as possible. Cases involving ingestion of more than one toxic species in which one set of symptoms masks or mimics another set are among many reasons for needing this information. Unfortunately, a number of factors (not discussed here) often make identification of the causative mushroom impossible. In such cases, diagnosis must be based on symptoms alone. In order to rule out other types of food poisoning and to conclude that the mushrooms eaten were the cause of the poisoning, it must be established that everyone who ate the suspect mushrooms became ill and that no one who did not eat the mushrooms became ill. Wild mushrooms eaten raw, cooked, or processed should always be regarded as prime suspects. After ruling out other sources of food poisoning and positively implicating mushrooms as the cause of the illness, diagnosis may proceed in two steps. The first step provides an early indication of the seriousness of the disease and its prognosis.

As described above, the protoplasmic poisons are the most likely to be fatal or to cause irreversible organ damage. In the case of poisoning by the deadly Amanitas, important laboratory indicators of liver (elevated LDH, SGOT, and bilirubin levels) and kidney (elevated uric acid, creatinine, and BUN levels) damage will be present. Unfortunately, in the absence of dietary history, these signs could be mistaken for symptoms of liver or kidney impairment as the result of other causes (e.g., viral hepatitis). It is important that this distinction be made as quickly as possible, because the delayed onset of symptoms will generally mean that the organ has already been damaged. The importance of rapid diagnosis is obvious: victims who are hospitalized and given aggressive support therapy almost immediately after ingestion have a mortality rate of only 10%, whereas those admitted 60 or more hours after ingestion have a 50–90% mortality rate. A recent report indicates that amanitins are observable in urine well before the onset of any symptoms, but that laboratory tests for liver dysfunction do not appear until well after the organ has been damaged.

6. Associated Foods

Mushroom poisonings are almost always caused by ingestion of wild mushrooms that have been collected by nonspecialists (although specialists have also been poisoned). Most cases occur when toxic species are confused with edible species, and a useful question to ask of the victims or their mushroom-picking benefactors is the identity of the mushroom they thought they were picking. In the absence of a well- preserved specimen, the answer to this question could narrow the possible suspects considerably. Intoxication has also occurred when reliance was placed on some folk method of distinguishing poisonous and safe species. Outbreaks have occurred after ingestion of fresh, raw mushrooms, stir-fried mushrooms, home-canned mushrooms, mushrooms cooked in tomato sauce (which rendered the sauce itself toxic, even when no mushrooms were consumed), and mushrooms that were blanched and frozen at home. Cases of poisoning by home-canned and frozen mushrooms are especially insidious because a single outbreak may easily become a multiple outbreak when the preserved toadstools are carried to another location and consumed at another time.

Specific cases of mistaken mushroom identity appear frequently. The Early False Morel *Gyromitra esculenta* is easily confused with the true Morel *Morchella esculenta,* and poisonings have occurred after consumption of fresh or cooked *Gyromitra. Gyromitra* poisonings have also occurred after ingestion of commercially available "morels" contaminated with *G. esculenta.* The commercial sources for these fungi (which have not yet been successfully cultivated on a large scale) are field collection of wild morels by semiprofessionals. Cultivated commercial mushrooms of whatever species are almost never implicated in poisoning outbreaks unless there are associated problems such as improper canning (which leads to bacterial food poisoning). Producers of mild gastroenteritis are too numerous to list here, but include members of many of the most abundant genera, including *Agaricus, Boletus, Lactarius, Russula, Tricholoma, Coprinus, Pluteus,* and others. The Inky Cap Mushroom *(Coprinus atrimentarius)* is considered both edible and delicious, and only the unwary who consume alcohol after eating this mushroom need be concerned. Some other members of the genus *Coprinus* (Shaggy Mane, *C. comatus;* Glistening Inky

Cap, *C. micaceus,* and others) and some of the larger
members of the *Lepiota* family such as the Parasol
Mushroom *(Leucocoprinus procera)* do not contain
coprine and do not cause this effect. The potentially
deadly Sorrel Webcap Mushroom *(Cortinarius orellanus)* is not easily distinguished from nonpoisonous
webcaps belonging to the same distinctive genus,
and all should be avoided.

Most of the psychotropic mushrooms (*Inocybe* spp.,
Conocybe spp., *Paneolus* spp., *Pluteus* spp.) are in general appearance small, brown, and leathery (the so-
called "Little Brown Mushrooms" or LBMs) and relatively unattractive from a culinary standpoint. The
Sweat Mushroom *(Clitocybe dealbata)* and the
Smoothcap Mushroom *(Psilocybe cubensis)* are small,
white, and leathery. These small, unattractive mushrooms are distinctive, fairly unappetizing, and not
easily confused with the fleshier fungi normally considered edible. Intoxications associated with them
are less likely to be accidental, although both *C. dealbata* and *Paneolus foenisicii* have been found growing
in the same fairy ring area as the edible (and choice)
Fairy Ring Mushroom *(Marasmius oreades)* and the
Honey Mushroom *(Armillariella mellea),* and have
been consumed when the picker has not carefully
examined every mushroom picked from the ring.
Psychotropic mushrooms, which are larger and
therefore more easily confused with edible mushrooms, include the Showy Flamecap or Big Laughing
Mushroom *(Gymnopilus spectabilis),* which has been
mistaken for Chanterelles *(Cantharellus* spp.) and for
Gymnopilus ventricosus found growing on wood of
conifers in western North America. The Fly Agaric
(Amanita muscaria) and Panthercap *(Amanita pantherina)* mushrooms are large, fleshy, and colorful.
Yellowish cap colors on some varieties of the Fly
Agaric and the Panthercap are similar to the edible
Caesar's Mushroom *(Amanita caesarea),* which is considered a delicacy in Italy. Another edible yellow
capped mushroom occasionally confused with yellow *A. muscaria* and *A. pantherina* varieties are the
Yellow Blusher *(Amanita flavorubens).* Orange to yel-
low-orange *A. muscaria* and *A. pantherina* may also be
confused with the Blusher *(Amanita rubescens)* and
the Honey Mushroom *(Armillariella mellea).* White to

pale forms of *A. muscaria* may be confused with edible field mushrooms (*Agaricus* spp.). Young (button stage) specimens of *A. muscaria* have also been confused with puffballs.

7. Relative Frequency of Disease

Accurate figures on the relative frequency of mushroom poisonings are difficult to obtain. For the 5-year period between 1976 and 1981, 16 outbreaks involving 44 cases were reported to the Centers for Disease Control in Atlanta (Rattanvilay et al. MMWR 31(21): 287–288, 1982). The number of unreported cases is, of course, unknown. Cases are sporadic and large outbreaks are rare. Poisonings tend to be grouped in the spring and fall when most mushroom species are at the height of their fruiting stage. While the actual incidence appears to be very low, the potential exists for grave problems. Poisonous mushrooms are not limited in distribution as are other poisonous organisms (such as dinoflagellates). Intoxications may occur at any time and place, with dangerous species occurring in habitats ranging from urban lawns to deep woods. As Americans become more adventurous in their mushroom collection and consumption, poisonings are likely to increase.

8. Target Population

All humans are susceptible to mushroom toxins. The poisonous species are ubiquitous, and geographical restrictions on types of poisoning that may occur in one location do not exist (except for some of the hallucinogenic LBMs, which occur primarily in the American southwest and southeast). Individual specimens of poisonous mushrooms are also characterized by individual variations in toxin content based on genetics, geographic location, and growing conditions. Intoxications may thus be more or less serious, depending not on the number of mushrooms consumed, but on the dose of toxin delivered. In addition, although most cases of poisoning by higher plants occur in children, toxic mushrooms are consumed most often by adults. Occasional accidental mushroom poisonings of children and pets have been reported, but adults are more likely to actively search for and consume wild mushrooms for culinary purposes. Children are more seriously affected by the normally nonlethal toxins than are adults and are more likely to suffer very serious consequences from ingestion of relatively smaller doses. Adults who consume mushrooms are also more likely to recall what was eaten and when, and are able to describe their symptoms more accurately than are children. Very old, very young, and debilitated persons of both sexes are more likely to become seriously ill from all types of mushroom poisoning, even those types which are generally considered to be mild.

Many idiosyncratic adverse reactions to mushrooms have been reported. Some mushrooms cause certain people to become violently ill, while not affecting others who consumed part of the same mushroom cap. Factors such as age, sex, and general health of the consumer do not seem to be reliable predictors of these reactions, and they have been attributed to allergic or hypersensitivity reactions and to inherited inability of the unfortunate victim to metabolize certain unusual fungal constituents (such as the uncommon sugar, trehalose). These reactions are probably not true poisonings as the general population does not seem to be affected.

9. Analysis of Foods for Toxins

The mushroom toxins can with difficulty be recovered from poisonous fungi, cooking water, stomach contents, serum, and urine. Procedures for extraction and quantitation are generally elaborate and time-consuming, and the patient will in most cases have recovered by the time an analysis is made on the basis of toxin chemistry. The exact chemical natures of most of the toxins that produce milder symptoms are unknown. Chromatographic techniques (TLC, GLC, HPLC) exist for the amanitins, orellanine, muscimol/ibotenic acid, psilocybin, muscarine, and the gyromitrins. The amanitins may also be determined by commercially available 3H-RIA kits. The most reliable means of diagnosing a mushroom poisoning remains botanical identification of the fungus that was eaten. An accurate pre-ingestion determination of species will also prevent accidental poisoning in 100% of cases. Accurate post-ingestion analyses for specific toxins when no botanical identification is possible may be essential only in cases of suspected poisoning by the deadly *Amanitas,* since prompt and aggressive therapy (including lavage, activated charcoal, and plasmapheresis) can greatly reduce the mortality rate.

10. Selected Outbreaks

Isolated cases of mushroom poisoning have occurred throughout the continental United States. One occurred in Oregon in October, 1988, and involved the intoxication of five people who consumed stir-fried *Amanita phalloides*. The poisonings were severe, and at this writing three of the five people had undergone liver transplants for treatment of amanitin-induced liver failure. Other recent cases have included the July, 1986, poisoning of a family in Philadelphia, by *Chlorophyllum molybdites*; the September, 1987, intoxication of seven men in Bucks County, PA, by spaghetti sauce which contained Jack O'Lantern mushroom *(Omphalotus illudens);* and of 14 teenage campers in Maryland by the same species (July, 1987). A report of a North Carolina outbreak of poisoning by False Morel (*Gyromitra* spp.) appeared in 1986. A 1985 report details a case of *Chlorophyllum molybdites* which occurred in Arkansas; a fatal poisoning case caused by an amanitin containing *Lepiota* was described in 1986. In 1981, two Berks County, PA, people were poisoned (one fatally) after ingesting *Amanita phalloides*, while in the same year, seven Laotian refugees living in California were poisoned by *Russula* spp. In separate 1981 incidents, several people from New York State were poisoned *by Omphalotus illudens, Amanita muscaria, Entoloma lividum,* and *Amanita virosa*. An outbreak of gastroenteritis during a banquet for 482 people in Vancouver, British Columbia, was reported by the Vancouver Health Department in June, 1991. Seventy-seven of the guests reported symptoms consisting of early onset nausea (15–30 min), diarrhea (20 min–13 hours), vomiting (20–60 min), cramps and bloated feeling. Other symptoms included feeling warm, clamminess, numbness of the tongue and extreme thirst along with two cases of hive-like rash with onset of 3–7 days. Bacteriological tests were negative. This intoxication merits special attention because it involved consumption of species normally considered not only edible but choice. The fungi involved were the morels *Morchella esculenta* and *M. elata (M. angusticeps),* which were prepared in a marinade and consumed raw. The symptoms were severe but not life threatening. Scattered reports of intoxications by these species and *M. conica* have appeared in anecdotal reports for many years.

Numerous other cases exist; however, the cases that appear in the literature tend to be the serious poisonings such as those causing more severe gastrointestinal symptoms, psychotropic reactions, and severe organ damage (deadly *Amanita*). Mild intoxications are probably grossly underreported, because of the lack of severity of symptoms and the unlikeliness of a hospital admission.

For more information on recent outbreaks see the *Morbidity and Mortality Weekly Reports* from CDC.

Aflatoxins

1. Name of Toxin

Aflatoxins

2. Name of Acute Disease

Aflatoxicosis

Aflatoxicosis is poisoning that results from ingestion of aflatoxins in contaminated food or feed. The aflatoxins are a group of structurally related toxic compounds produced by certain strains of the fungi *Aspergillus flavus* and *A. parasiticus*. Under favorable conditions of temperature and humidity, these fungi grow on certain foods and feeds, resulting in the production of aflatoxins. The most pronounced contamination has been encountered in tree nuts, peanuts, and other oilseeds, including corn and cottonseed. The major aflatoxins of concern are designated B1, B2, G1, and G2. These toxins are usually found together in various foods and feeds in various proportions; however, aflatoxin B1 is usually predominant and is the most toxic. When a commodity is analyzed by thin-layer chromatography, the aflatoxins separate into the individual components in the order given above; however, the first two fluoresce blue when viewed under ultraviolet light and the second two fluoresce green. Aflatoxin M is a major metabolic product of aflatoxin B1 in animals and is usually excreted in the milk and urine of dairy cattle and other mammalian species that have consumed aflatoxin-contaminated food or feed.

3. Nature of Disease

Aflatoxins produce acute necrosis, cirrhosis, and carcinoma of the liver in a number of animal species; no animal species is resistant to the acute toxic effects of aflatoxins; hence it is logical to assume that humans may be similarly affected. A wide variation in LD50 values has been obtained in animal species tested with single doses of aflatoxins. For most species, the LD50 value ranges from 0.5 to 10 mg/kg body weight. Animal species respond differently in their susceptibility to the chronic and acute toxicity of aflatoxins. The toxicity can be influenced by environmental factors, exposure level, and duration of exposure, age, health, and nutritional status of diet. Aflatoxin B1 is a very potent carcinogen in many species, including nonhuman primates, birds, fish, and rodents. In each species, the liver is the primary target organ of acute injury. Metabolism plays a major role in determining the toxicity of aflatoxin B1; studies show that this aflatoxin requires metabolic activation to exert its carcinogenic effect, and these effects can be modified by induction or inhibition of the mixed function oxidase system.

4. Normal Course of Disease

In well-developed countries, aflatoxin contamination rarely occurs in foods at levels that cause acute aflatoxicosis in humans. In view of this, studies on human toxicity from ingestion of aflatoxins have focused on their carcinogenic potential. The relative susceptibility of humans to aflatoxins is not known, even though epidemiological studies in Africa and Southeast Asia, where there is a high incidence of hepatoma, have revealed an association between cancer incidence and the aflatoxin content of the diet. These studies have not proved a cause-effect relationship, but the evidence suggests an association.

One of the most important accounts of aflatoxicosis in humans occurred in more than 150 villages in adjacent districts of two neighboring states in northwest India in the fall of 1974. According to one report of this outbreak, 397 persons were affected and 108 persons died. In this outbreak, contaminated corn was the major dietary constituent, and aflatoxin levels of 0.25 to 15 mg/kg were found. The daily aflatoxin B1 intake was estimated to have been at least 55 ug/kg body weight for an undetermined number of days. The patients experienced high fever, rapid progressive jaundice, edema of the limbs, pain, vomiting, and swollen livers. One investigator reported a peculiar and very notable feature of the outbreak: the appearance of signs of disease in one village population was preceded by a similar disease in domestic dogs, which was usually fatal. Histopathological examination of humans showed extensive bile duct proliferation and periportal fibrosis of the liver together with gastrointestinal hemorrhages. A 10-year follow-up of the Indian outbreak found the survivors fully recovered with no ill effects from the experience.

A second outbreak of aflatoxicosis was reported from Kenya in 1982. There were 20 hospital admissions with a 60% mortality; daily aflatoxin intake was estimated to be at least 38 ug/kg body weight for an undetermined number of days.

In a deliberate suicide attempt, a laboratory worker ingested 12 ug/kg body weight of aflatoxin B1 per day over a 2-day period and 6 months later, 11 ug/kg body weight per day over a 14-day period. Except for transient rash, nausea and headache, there were no ill effects; hence, these levels may serve as possible no-effect levels for aflatoxin B1 in humans. In a 14-year follow-up, a physical examination and blood chemistry, including tests for liver function, were normal.

5. Diagnosis of Human Illnesses

Aflatoxicosis in humans has rarely been reported; however, such cases are not always recognized. Aflatoxicosis may be suspected when a disease outbreak exhibits the following characteristics:
- the cause is not readily identifiable
- the condition is not transmissible
- syndromes may be associated with certain batches of food
- treatment with antibiotics or other drugs has little effect
- the outbreak may be seasonal, i.e., weather conditions may affect mold growth.

The adverse effects of aflatoxins in animals (and presumably in humans) have been categorized in two general forms.

A. (Primary) Acute aflatoxicosis is produced when moderate to high levels of aflatoxins are consumed. Specific, acute episodes of disease ensue and may include hemorrhage, acute liver damage, edema, alteration in digestion, absorption and/or metabolism of nutrients, and possibly death.

B. (Primary) Chronic aflatoxicosis results from ingestion of low to moderate levels of aflatoxins. The effects are usually subclinical and difficult to recognize. Some of the common symptoms are impaired food conversion and slower rates of growth with or without the production of an overt aflatoxin syndrome.

6. Associated Foods

In the United States, aflatoxins have been identified in corn and corn products, peanuts and peanut products, cottonseed, milk, and tree nuts such as Brazil nuts, pecans, pistachio nuts, and walnuts. Other grains and nuts are susceptible but less prone to contamination.

7. Relative Frequency of Disease

The relative frequency of aflatoxicosis in humans in the United States is not known. No outbreaks have been reported in humans. Sporadic cases have been reported in animals.

8. Target Populations

Although humans and animals are susceptible to the effects of acute aflatoxicosis, the chance of human exposure to acute levels of aflatoxin is remote in well-developed countries. In undeveloped countries, human susceptibility can vary with age, health, and level and duration of exposure.

9. Analysis of Foods

Many chemical procedures have been developed to identify and measure aflatoxins in various commodities. The basic steps include extraction, lipid removal, cleanup, separation and quantification. Depending on the nature of the commodity, methods can sometimes be simplified by omitting unnecessary steps. Chemical methods have been developed for peanuts, corn, cottonseed, various tree nuts, and animal feeds. Chemical methods for aflatoxin in milk and dairy products are far more sensitive than for the above commodities because the aflatoxin M animal metabolite is usually found at much lower levels (ppb and ppt). All collaboratively studied methods for aflatoxin analysis are described in Chapter 26 of the AOAC Official Methods of Analysis.

10. Outbreaks

Very little information is available on outbreaks of aflatoxicosis in humans because medical services are less developed in the areas of the world where high levels of contamination of aflatoxins occur in foods, and, therefore, many cases go unnoticed.

For more information on recent outbreaks see the *Morbidity and Mortality Weekly Reports* from CDC.

The Center for Science in the Public Interest (CSPI) is a nonprofit organization concerned with improving human health through better nutrition and food safety. This report, "Chemical Cuisine," first appeared in *Nutrition Action Healthletter,* the center's newsletter on food and health issues. The food additives listed are among the most frequently added to food. Additives are listed alphabetically, and symbols indicate which are safe to consume, which should be consumed with caution, and which should be avoided. The table at the end shows banned additives and the reasons they were banned. This may be viewed online at http://www.cspinet.org/reports/chemcuisine.htm.

Chemical Cuisine: CSPI's Guide to Food Additives

Introduction to Food Additives

Shopping was easy when most food came from farms. Now, factory-made foods have made chemical additives a significant part of our diet. Most people may not be able to pronounce the names of many of these chemicals, but they still want to know what the chemicals do and which ones are safe and which are poorly tested or possibly dangerous. This listing provides that information for most common additives. A simple general rule about additives is to avoid sodium nitrite, saccharin, caffeine, olestra, acesulfame-K, and artificial coloring. Not only are they among the most questionable additives, but they are used primarily in foods of low nutritional value. Also, don't forget the two most familiar additives: sugar and salt. They may pose the greatest risk because we consume so much of them. Fortunately, most additives are safe and some even increase the nutritional value of the food. Additional information about some of the additives is available elsewhere in this Web site. Use the search engine provided to locate that information.

Glossary

ANTIOXIDANTS retard the oxidation of unsaturated fats and oils, colorings, and flavorings. Oxidation leads to rancidity, flavor changes, and loss of color. Most of those effects are caused by reaction of oxygen in the air with fats.

CARCINOGEN is a chemical or other agent that causes cancer in animals or humans.

CHELATING AGENTS trap trace amounts of metal atoms that would otherwise cause food to discolor or go rancid.

EMULSIFIERS keep oil and water mixed together.

FLAVOR ENHANCERS have little or no flavor of their own, but accentuate the natural flavor of foods. They are often used when very little of a natural ingredient is present.

THICKENING AGENTS are natural or chemically modified carbohydrates that absorb some of the water that is present in food, thereby making the food thicker. Thickening agents "stabilize" factory-made foods by keeping the complex mixtures of oils, water, acids, and solids well mixed.

Cancer Testing

Chemicals usually are tested for an ability to cause cancer by feeding large dosages to small numbers of rats and mice. Large dosages are used to compensate for the small number of animals that can be used (a few hundred is considered a big study, though it is tiny compared to the U.S. population of 270 million). Also, the large dosages can compensate for the possibility that rodents may be less sensitive than people to a particular chemical (as happened with thalidomide). Some people claim that such tests are improper and that large amounts of any chemical would cause cancer.

That is not true. Huge amounts of most chemicals do not cause cancer. When a large dosage causes cancer, most scientists believe that a smaller amount would also cause cancer, but less frequently. It would be nice if lower, more realistic dosages could be used, but a test using low dosages and a small number of animals would be extraordinarily insensitive. It would also be nice if test-tube tests not using any animals were developed that could cheaply and accurately identify cancer-causing chemicals. While some progress has been made in that direction, those tests have not proven reliable. Thus, the standard high-dosage cancer test on small numbers of animals is currently the only practical, reasonably reliable way to identify food additives (and other chemicals) that might cause cancer.

The Delaney Clause is an important part of the federal Food, Drug, and Cosmetic Act. That important consumer-protection clause specifically bans any additive that "is found to induce cancer when ingested by man or animal." The food and chemical industries are seeking to weaken or repeal that law.

Alphabetical Listing of Additives

✓ Safe. The additive appears to be safe.

✂ Cut back on this. Not toxic, but large amounts may be unsafe or promote bad nutrition.

✕ Caution. May pose a risk and needs to be better tested. Try to avoid.

▲ Certain people should avoid these additives.

⊘ Everyone should avoid. Unsafe in amounts consumed or is very poorly tested and not worth any risk.

⊘ ACESULFAME-K . . . Artificial sweetener: Baked goods, chewing gum, gelatin desserts, soft drinks.

This artificial sweetener, manufactured by Hoechst, a giant German chemical company, is widely used around the world. It is about 200 times sweeter than sugar. In the United States, for several years acesulfame-K (the K is the chemical symbol for potassium) was permitted only in such foods as sugar-free baked goods, chewing gum, and gelatin desserts. In July 1998, the FDA allowed this chemical to be used in soft drinks, thereby greatly increasing consumer exposure.

The safety tests of acesulfame-K were conducted in the 1970s and were of mediocre quality. Key rat tests were afflicted by disease in the animal colonies; a mouse study was several months too brief and did not expose animals during gestation. Two rat studies suggest that the additive might cause cancer. It was for those reasons that in 1996 the Center for Science in the Public Interest urged the FDA to require better testing before permitting acesulfame-K in soft drinks. In addition, large doses of ace-toacetamide, a breakdown product, have been shown to affect the thyroid in rats, rabbits, and dogs. Hopefully, the small amounts in food are not harmful.

✓ ALGINATE, PROPYLENE GLYCOL ALGINATE . . . Thickening agents, foam stabilizer: Ice cream, cheese, candy, yogurt.

Alginate, an apparently safe derivative of seaweed (kelp), maintains the desired texture in dairy products, canned frosting, and other factory-made foods Propylene glycol alginate, chemically-modified algin, thickens acidic foods (soda pop, salad dressing) and can stabilize the foam in beer.

✓ ALPHA TOCOPHEROL (Vitamin E) . . . Antioxidant, nutrient: Vegetable oil.

Vitamin E is abundant in whole wheat, rice germ, and vegetable oils. It is destroyed by the refining and bleaching of flour.

Vitamin E prevents oils from going rancid. Recent studies indicate that large amounts of vitamin E may help reduce the risk of heart disease and cancer.

ARTIFICIAL COLORINGS.

Most artificial colorings are synthetic chemicals that do not occur in nature. Because colorings are used almost solely in foods of low nutritional value (candy, soda pop, gelatin desserts, etc.), you should simply avoid all artificially colored foods. In addition to problems mentioned below, colorings cause hyperactivity in some sensitive children. The use of coloring usually indicates that fruit or other natural ingredient has not been used.

• ⊘ BLUE 1 . . . Artificial coloring: Beverages, candy, baked goods.

Inadequately tested; suggestions of a small cancer risk.

• ⊘ BLUE 2 . . . Artificial coloring: Pet food, beverages, candy.

The largest study suggested, but did not prove, that this dye caused brain tumors in male mice. The FDA concluded that there is "reasonable certainty of no harm."

- ✗   CITRUS RED 2 ... Artificial coloring: Skin of some Florida oranges only.

  Studies indicated that this additive causes cancer. The dye does not seep through the orange skin into the pulp. No risk except when eating peel.

- ⊘   GREEN 3 ... Artificial colorings: Candy, beverages.

  A 1981 industry-sponsored study gave hints of bladder cancer, but FDA re-analyzed the data using other statistical tests and concluded that the dye was safe. Fortunately, this possibly carcinogenic dye is rarely used.

- ⊘   RED 3 ... Artificial coloring: Cherries in fruit cocktail, candy, baked goods.

  The evidence that this dye caused thyroid tumors in rats is "convincing," according to 1983 review committee report requested by FDA. FDA's recommendation that the dye be banned was overruled by pressure from elsewhere in the Reagan Administration.

- ✗   RED 40 ... Artificial coloring: Soda pop, candy, gelatin desserts, pastry, pet food, sausage.

  The most widely used food dye. While this is one of the most-tested food dyes, the key mouse tests were flawed and inconclusive. An FDA review committee acknowledged problems, but said evidence of harm was not "consistent" or "substantial." Like other dyes, Red 40 is used mainly in junk foods.

- ▲   YELLOW 5 ... Artificial coloring: Gelatin dessert, candy, pet food, baked goods.

  The second most widely used coloring causes mild allergic reactions, primarily in aspirin-sensitive persons.

- ⊘   YELLOW 6 ... Artificial coloring: Beverages, sausage, baked goods, candy, gelatin.

  Industry-sponsored animal tests indicated that this dye, the third most widely used, causes tumors of the adrenal gland and kidney. In addition, small amounts of several carcinogen contaminate Yellow 6. However, the FDA reviewed those data and found reasons to conclude that Yellow 6 does not pose a significant cancer risk to humans. Yellow 6 may also cause occasional allergic reactions.

ARTIFICIAL AND NATURAL FLAVORING . . . Flavoring: Soda pop, candy, breakfast cereals, gelatin desserts, and many other foods.

Hundreds of chemicals are used to mimic natural flavors; many may be used in a single flavoring, such as for cherry soda pop. Most flavoring chemicals also occur in nature and are probably safe, but they are used almost exclusively in junk foods. Their use indicates that the real thing (often fruit) has been left out. Companies keep the identity of artificial (and natural) flavorings a deep secret. Flavorings may include substances to which some people are sensitive, such as MSG or HVP.

✓ ASCORBIC ACID (Vitamin C), SODIUM ASCORBATE . . . Antioxidant, unwanted nutrient, color stabilizer: Cereals, fruit drinks, cured meats.

Ascorbic acid helps maintain the red color of cured meat and prevents the formation of nitrosamines, which promote cancer (see SODIUM NITRITE). It helps prevent loss of color and flavor by reacting with oxygen. It is used as a nutrient additive in drinks and cereals. Sodium ascorbate is a more soluble form of ascorbic acid. ERYTHORBIC ACID is very similar to ascorbic acid, but has no value as a vitamin. Large amounts of ascorbic acid may reduce the severity of colds and offer other health benefits.

✗ ▲ ASPARTAME . . . Artificial sweetener: "Diet" foods, including soft drinks, drink mixes, gelatin desserts, low-calorie frozen desserts, packets.

Aspartame (Equal, NutraSweet), made up primarily of two amino acids, was thought to be the perfect artificial sweetener, but questions have arisen about the quality of the cancer tests, which should be repeated. Some persons have reported adverse behavioral effects (dizziness, hallucinations, headache) after drinking diet soda, but such reports have not been confirmed in controlled studies. If you think you've experienced adverse effects due to aspartame, avoid it. Also, people with the rare disease PKU (phenylketonuria) need to avoid it. There is little evidence that this or other artificial sweeteners have helped people lose weight, though those additives might help some strong-willed dieters.

Indeed, since 1980, consumption of artificial sweeteners and rates of obesity have both soared.

✓ BETA-CAROTENE . . . Coloring; nutrient: Margarine, shortening, non-dairy whiteners.

Beta-carotene is used as an artificial coloring and a nutrient supplement. The body converts it to Vitamin A, which is part of the light-detection mechanism of the eye and which helps maintain the normal condition of mucous membranes. Large dietary supplements increased the risk of lung cancer in smokers and did not reduce the risk in non-smokers. Smokers should certainly not take beta-carotene supplements, but the small amounts used as food additives are safe.

✗ BROMINATED VEGETABLE OIL (BVO) . . . Emulsifier, clouding agent: Soft drinks.

BVO keeps flavor oils in suspension and gives a cloudy appearance to citrus-flavored soft drinks. Eating BVO leaves small residues in body fat; it is unclear whether those residues pose any risk. Fortunately, BVO is not widely used.

✗ BUTYLATED HYDROXY-ANISOLE (BHA) . . . Antioxidant: Cereals, chewing gum, potato chips, vegetable oil.

BHA retards rancidity in fats, oils, and oil-containing foods. While most studies indicate it is safe, some studies demonstrated that it caused cancer in rats. This synthetic chemical can be replaced by safer chemicals (e.g., vitamin E), safer processes (e.g., packing foods under nitrogen instead of air), or can simply be left out (many brands of oily foods, such as potato chips, don't use any antioxidant).

✗ BUTYLATED HYDROXYTOLUENE (BHT) . . . Antioxidant: Cereals, chewing gum, potato chips, oils, etc.

BHT retards rancidity in oils. It either increased or decreased the risk of cancer in various animal studies. Residues of BHT occur in human fat. BHT is unnecessary or is easily replaced by safe substitutes (see discussion of BHA). Avoid it when possible.

✗ ✂ CAFFEINE . . . Stimulant: Naturally occurring in

Caffeine is the only drug that is present naturally or added to widely consumed foods (quinine is the other drug used in foods). It is mildly addictive, one possible coffee, tea, cocoa, coffee-flavored yogurt and frozen desserts. Additive in soft drinks, gum, and waters.

reason that makers of soft drinks add it to their products. Many coffee drinkers experience withdrawal symptoms, such as headaches, irritability, sleepiness, and lethargy, when they stop drinking coffee. Because caffeine increases the risk of miscarriages (and possibly birth defects) and inhibits fetal growth, it should be avoided by women who are pregnant or considering becoming pregnant. It also may make it harder to get pregnant (but don't use it as a birth-control pill!). Caffeine also keeps many people from sleeping, causes jitteriness, and affects calcium metabolism. The caffeine in a cup or two of coffee is harmless to most people. But if you drink more than a couple of cups of coffee or cans of caffeine-containing soda per day, experience symptoms noted above, are at risk of osteoporosis, or are pregnant, you should rethink your habit.

✓ CALCIUM (or SODIUM) PROPIONATE . . . Preservative: Bread, rolls, pies, cakes.

Calcium propionate prevents mold growth on bread and rolls. The calcium is a beneficial mineral; the propionate is safe. Sodium propionate is used in pies and cakes, because calcium alters the action of chemical leavening agents.

✓ CALCIUM (or SODIUM) STEAROYL LACTYLATE . . . Dough conditioner, whipping agent: Bread dough, cake fillings, artificial whipped cream, processed egg whites.

These additives strengthen bread dough so it can be used in bread-making machinery and help produce a more uniform grain and greater volume. They act as whipping agents in dried, liquid, or frozen egg whites and artificial whipped cream. SODIUM STEAROYL FUMARATE serves the same function.

▲ CARMINE; COCHINEAL EXTRACT . . . Artificial coloring.

Cochineal extract is a coloring extracted from the eggs of the cochineal beetle, which lives on cactus plants in Peru, the Canary Islands, and elsewhere. Carmine is a more purified coloring made from cochineal. In both cases, the actual substance that provides the color is carminic acid. These colorings, which are extremely stable, are used in some red, pink, or purple candy, yogurt, Campari, ice cream, beverages, and many other foods, as well as drugs and cosmetics. These colorings have caused allergic reactions that range from hives to life-threatening anaphylactic shock. It is not known how many people suffer from this allergy. The Food and Drug Administration should ban cochineal extract and carmine or, at the very least, require that they be identified clearly on food labels so that people could avoid them. Natural or synthetic substitutes are available. A label statement should also disclose that Carmine is extracted from dried insects so that vegetarians and others who want to avoid animal products could do so.

✓ CARRAGEENAN . . . Thickening and stabilizing agent: Ice cream, jelly, chocolate milk, infant formula.

Carrageenan is obtained from seaweed. Large amounts of carrageenan have harmed test animals' colons; the small amounts in food are safe.

▲ CASEIN, SODIUM CASEINATE . . . Thickening and whitening agent: Ice cream, ice milk, sherbet, coffee creamers.

Casein, the principal protein in milk, is a nutritious protein containing adequate amounts of all the essential amino acids. People who are allergic to casein should read food labels carefully, because the additive is used in some "non-dairy" and "vegetarian" foods.

✓ CITRIC ACID, SODIUM CITRATE . . . Acid, flavoring, chelating agent: Ice cream, sherbet, fruit drink, candy, carbonated beverages, instant potatoes.

Citric acid is versatile, widely used, cheap, and safe. It is an important metabolite in virtually all living organisms and is abundant naturally in citrus fruits and berries. It is used as a strong acid, a tart flavoring, and an antioxidant. Sodium citrate, also safe, is a buffer that controls the acidity of gelatin desserts, jam, and other foods.

COCHINEAL EXTRACT. *See* CARMINE.

✄ CORN SYRUP . . . Sweetener, thickener: Candy,

Corn syrup, which consists mostly of dextrose, is a sweet, thick liquid made by treating cornstarch with acids or enzymes. It toppings, syrups, snack foods, imitation dairy foods.

may be dried and used as corn syrup solids in coffee whiteners and other dry products. Corn syrup contains no nutritional value other than calories, promotes tooth decay, and is used mainly in foods with little intrinsic nutritional value.

⊘ CYCLAMATE . . . Artificial sweetener: Diet foods.

This controversial high-potency sweetener was used in the United States in diet foods until 1970, at which time it was banned. Animal studies indicated that it causes cancer. Now, based on animal studies, it (or a by-product) is believed not to cause cancer directly, but to increase the potency of other carcinogens and to harm the testes.

 DEXTROSE (GLUCOSE, CORN SUGAR) . . . Sweetener, coloring agent: Bread, caramel, soda pop, cookies, many other foods.

Dextrose is an important chemical in every living organism. A sugar, it is a source of sweetness in fruits and honey. Added to foods as a sweetener, it represents empty calories and contributes to tooth decay. Dextrose turns brown when heated and contributes to the color of bread crust and toast. Americans consume about 25 pounds per year of dextrose—and a total of about 150 pounds per year of all refined sugars.

✓ EDTA . . . Chelating agent: Salad dressing, margarine, sandwich spreads, mayonnaise, processed fruits and vegetables, canned shellfish, soft drinks.

Modern food-manufacturing technology, which involves rollers, blenders, and containers made of metal, results in trace amounts of metal contamination in food. EDTA (ethylenediamine tetraacetic acid) traps metal impurities, which would otherwise promote rancidity and the breakdown of artificial colors. It is safe.

✓ ERYTHORBIC ACID . . . Antioxidant, color stabilizer: Cured meats. See ASCORBIC ACID.

✓ FERROUS GLUCONATE . . . Coloring, nutrient: Black olives.

Used by the olive industry to generate a uniform jet-black color and in pills as a source of iron. Safe.

✓ FOOD-STARCH,
MODIFIED. See
STARCH, MODIFIED
below.

✓ FUMARIC ACID . . .   A solid at room temperature, inexpensive,
Tartness agent: highly acidic, fumaric acid is the ideal
Powdered drinks,   source of tartness and acidity in dry food
pudding, pie   products. However, it dissolves slowly in
fillings, gelatin   cold water, a drawback cured by adding
desserts.   DIOCTYL SODIUM SULFOSUCCINATE (DSS), a
detergent-like additive that appears to be
safe.

✓ GELATIN . . .   Gelatin is a protein obtained from animal
Thickening and   hides and bones. It has little nutritional
gelling agent: value because it contains little or none of
Powdered dessert   several essential amino acids.
mixes, yogurt, ice
cream, cheese
spreads, beverages.

✓ GLYCERIN (GLYCEROL)   In nature, glycerin forms the backbone of fat
. . . Maintains   and oil molecules. The body uses it as a
water content: source of energy or as a starting material in
Marshmallows,   making more-complex molecules.
candy, fudge,
baked goods.

✓ ▲ GUMS: Arabic,   Gums are derived from natural sources
Furcelleran,   (bushes, trees, seaweed, bacteria) and are
Ghatti, Guar,   poorly tested, though probably safe. They
Karaya, Locust   are not absorbed by the body. They are used
Bean, Tragacanth,   to thicken foods, prevent sugar crystals
Xanthan . . .   from forming in candy, stabilize beer foam
Thickening   (arabic), form a gel in pudding (furcelleran),
agents,   encapsulate flavor oils in powdered drink
stabilizers: mixes, or keep oil and water mixed together
Beverages, ice   in salad dressings. Gums are often used to
cream, frozen   replace fat in low-fat ice cream, baked
pudding, salad   goods, and salad dressings. Tragacanth has
dressing, dough,   caused occasional severe allergic reactions.
cottage cheese,
candy, drink
mixes.

X **HEPTYL PARABEN . . .** Heptyl paraben—short for the heptyl ester Preservative: Beer, of para-hydroxybenzoic acid—is a preserva- non-carbonated tive. Studies suggest that this rarely used soft drinks. additive chemical is safe, but it, like other additives in alcoholic beverages, has never been tested in the presence of alcohol (such as in animals weakened by long-term con- sumption of alcohol).

✂ **HIGH-FRUCTOSE** Corn syrup can be treated with enzymes to **CORN SYRUP . . .** convert some of its dextrose to fructose, Sweetener: Soft which results in High Fructose Corn Syrup drinks, other (HFCS). HFCS has largely replaced ordinary processed foods. sugar used in soft drinks and many other foods because it is cheaper. Americans con- sume about 59 pounds per year of HFCS (and a total of 150 pounds per year of all refined sugars).

✂ **HYDROGENATED** HSH, like sorbitol, is slightly sweet and **STARCH** poorly absorbed by the body. Like sorbitol, **HYDROLYSATE (HSH)** and other sugar alcohols, eating significant . . . Sweetener: amounts of HSH may cause intestinal gas Dietetic and and diarrhea. reduced-calorie foods.

✂ **HYDROGENATED** Vegetable oil, usually a liquid, can be made **VEGETABLE OIL,** into a semi-solid shortening by reacting it **PARTIALLY** with hydrogen. Hydrogenation reduces the **HYDROGENATED** levels of polyunsaturated oils—and also **VEGETABLE OIL . . .** creates trans fats, which promote heart Fat, oil, disease (they act like saturated fats). Ideally, shortening: food manufacturers would replace Margarine, hydrogenated shortening with less-harmful crackers, fried ingredients. restaurant foods, baked goods.

▲ **HYDROLYZED** HVP consists of vegetable (usually soybean) **VEGETABLE** protein that has been chemically broken **PROTEIN (HVP) . . .** down to the amino acids of which it is com- Flavor enhancer: posed. HVP is used to bring out the natural Instant soups, flavor of food (and, perhaps, to enable com-

frankfurters, sauce
mixes, beef stew.

panies to use less real food). It contains MSG
and may cause adverse reactions in sensitive individuals.

✂ INVERT SUGAR . . .
Sweetener: Candy,
soft drinks, many
other foods.

Invert sugar, a 50–50 mixture of two sugars,
dextrose and fructose, is sweeter and more
soluble than sucrose (table sugar). Invert
sugar forms when sucrose is split in two by
an enzyme or acid. It provides "empty calories," contributes to tooth decay, and should
be avoided.

✓ LACTIC ACID . . .
Controls acidity:
Spanish olives,
cheese, frozen
desserts,
carbonated
beverages.

This safe acid occurs in almost all living
organisms. It inhibits spoilage in Spanish-type olives, balances the acidity in cheese-making, and adds tartness to frozen
desserts, carbonated fruit-flavored drinks,
and other foods.

▲ LACTOSE . . .
Sweetener:
Whipped topping
mix, breakfast
pastry.

Lactose, a carbohydrate found only in milk,
is one of Nature's ways of delivering
calories to infant mammals. One-sixth as
sweet as table sugar, lactose is added to
food as a slightly sweet source of carbohydrate. Milk turns sour when bacteria convert lactose to lactic acid. Many people,
especially non-Caucasians, have trouble
digesting lactose. Bacteria in their guts may
produce gas.

✓ LECITHIN . . .
Emulsifier,
antioxidant: Baked
goods, margarine,
chocolate, ice cream.

A common constituent of animal and plant
tissues, lecithin is a source of the nutrient
choline. It keeps oil and water from separating out, retards rancidity, reduces spattering
in a frying pan, and leads to fluffier cakes.
Major natural sources are egg yolk and soybeans.

✂ MALTITOL . . .
Sweetener: Dietetic
and other reduced
calorie foods.

Like mannitol, sorbitol, and other sugar
alcohols, maltitol may be expected to promote flatulence and other gastrointestinal
symptoms.

✂ MANNITOL . . .
Sweetener, other
uses: Chewing

Not quite as sweet as sugar and poorly
absorbed by the body, it contributes only
half as many calories as sugar. Used as the

gum, low-calorie foods.

"dust" on chewing gum, mannitol prevents gum from absorbing moisture and becoming sticky. Safe—except that large amounts that are used in gum may have a laxative effect and even cause diarrhea.

 MONO- and DIGLYCERIDES ... Emulsifier: Baked goods, margarine, candy, peanut butter.

Makes bread softer and prevents staling, improves the stability of margarine, makes caramels less sticky, and prevents the oil in peanut butter from separating out. Mono- and diglycerides are safe, though most foods they are used in are high in refined flour, sugar, or fat.

▲ MONOSODIUM GLUTAMATE (MSG) ... Flavor enhancer: Soup, salad dressing, chips, frozen entrees, restaurant foods.

This amino acid brings out the flavor in many foods. While that may sound like a treat for taste buds, the use of MSG allows companies to reduce the amount of real ingredients in their foods, such as chicken in chicken soup. In the 1960s, it was discovered that large amounts of MSG fed to infant mice destroyed nerve cells in the brain. After that research was publicized, public pressure forced baby-food companies to stop adding MSG to their products (it was used to make the foods taste better to parents).

Careful studies have shown that some people are sensitive to MSG. Reactions include headache, nausea, weakness, and burning sensation in the back of neck and forearms. Some people complain of wheezing, changes in heart rate, and difficulty breathing. Some people claim to be sensitive to very small amounts of MSG, but no good studies have been done to determine just how little MSG can cause a reaction in the most-sensitive people. To protect the public's health, manufacturers and restaurateurs should use less or no MSG and the amounts of MSG should be listed on labels of foods that contain significant amounts. People who believe they are sensitive to MSG should be aware that other ingredients, such as natural flavoring and hydrolyzed vegetable protein, also contain glutamate. Also, foods such as

Parmesan cheese and tomatoes contain glutamate that occurs naturally, but no reactions have been reported to those foods.

✂ OLESTRA (Olean) . . .
Fat substitute:
Chips, crackers.

Olestra is Procter & Gamble's synthetic fat that is not absorbed by the body, but runs right through. Procter & Gamble suggests that replacing regular fat with olestra will help people lose weight and lower the risk of heart disease.

Olestra can cause diarrhea and loose stools, abdominal cramps, flatulence, and other adverse effects. Those symptoms are sometimes severe.

Even more importantly, olestra reduces the body's ability to absorb fat-soluble carotenoids (such as alpha and beta-carotene, lycopene, lutein, and canthaxanthin) from fruits and vegetables. Those nutrients are thought by many experts to reduce the risk of cancer and heart disease. Olestra enables manufacturers to offer greasy-feeling low-fat snacks, but consumers would be much better off with baked snacks, which are perfectly safe and just as low in calories. Products made with olestra should not be called "fat free," because they contain substantial amounts of indigestible fat.

✓ PHOSPHORIC ACID;
PHOSPHATES . . .
Acidulant,
chelating agent,
buffer, emulsifier,
nutrient, discoloration inhibitor:
Baked goods,
cheese, powdered
foods, cured meat,
soda pop, breakfast cereals,
dehydrated
potatoes.

Phosphoric acid acidifies and flavors cola beverages. CALCIUM and IRON PHOSPHATES act as mineral supplements. SODIUM ACID PYROPHOSPHATE is a leavening agent. CALCIUM and AMMONIUM PHOSPHATES serve as food for yeast in baking. SODIUM ACID PYROPHOSPHATE prevents discoloration in potatoes and sugar syrups. While excessive consumption of phosphates could lead to dietary imbalances that might contribute to osteoporosis, only a small fraction of the phosphate in the American diet comes from additives. Most comes from meat and dairy products.

✓ PLANT STEROL ESTERS . . . Cholesterol-lowering additive: Margarine, other foods.

These substances, which are extracted from pine trees, reduce the absorption of cholesterol from food and lower blood cholesterol levels. They are not toxic, but they may reduce the body's absorption of nutrients called carotenoids that are thought to reduce the risk of cancer and heart disease. Used in Benecol-brand products (margarine, salad dressing, and others).

✓ POLYSORBATE 60 . . . Emulsifier: Baked goods, frozen desserts, imitation dairy products.

Polysorbate 60 is short for polyoxyethylene-(20)-sorbitan monostearate. It and its close relatives, POLYSORBATE 65 and 80, work the same way as mono- and diglycerides, but smaller amounts are needed. They keep baked goods from going stale, keep dill oil dissolved in bottled dill pickles, help coffee whiteners dissolve in coffee, and prevent oil from separating out of artificial whipped cream.

⊘ POTASSIUM BROMATE . . . Flour improver: Bread and rolls.

This additive has long been used to increase the volume of bread and to produce bread with a fine crumb (the not-crust part of bread) structure. Most bromate rapidly breaks down to form innocuous bromide. However, bromate itself causes cancer in animals. The tiny amounts of bromate that may remain in bread pose a small risk to consumers. Bromate has been banned virtually worldwide except in Japan and the United States. It is rarely used in California because a cancer warning might be required on the label. In 1999, the Center for Science in the Public Interest petitioned the FDA to ban bromate.

⊘ PROPYL GALLATE . . . Antioxidant preservative: Vegetable oil, meat products, potato sticks, chicken soup base, chewing gum.

Propyl gallate retards the spoilage of fats and oils and is often used with BHA and BHT, because of the synergistic effects these preservatives have. The best studies on rats and mice were peppered with suggestions (but not proof) that this preservative might cause cancer. Avoid.

✕ ▲ QUININE . . .
Flavoring: Tonic
water, quinine
water, bitter
lemon.

This drug can cure malaria and is used as a bitter flavoring in a few soft drinks. There is a slight chance that quinine causes birth defects, so, to be on the safe side, pregnant women should avoid quinine-containing beverages and drugs. Relatively poorly tested.

⊘ SACCHARIN . . .
Artificial
sweetener:
"Diet" products,
soft drinks
(especially
fountain drinks at
restaurants),
packets.

Saccharin (Sweet 'N Low) is 350 times sweeter than sugar and is used in dietetic foods or as a tabletop sugar substitute. Many studies on animals have shown that saccharin can cause cancer of the urinary bladder. In other rodent studies, saccharin has caused cancer of the uterus, ovaries, skin, blood vessels, and other organs. Other studies have shown that saccharin increases the potency of other cancer-causing chemicals. And the best epidemiology study (done by the National Cancer Institute) found that the use of artificial sweeteners (saccharin and cyclamate) was associated with a higher incidence of bladder cancer.

In 1977, the FDA proposed that saccharin be banned, because of studies that it causes cancer in animals. However, Congress intervened and has permitted it to be used, provided that foods bear a warning notice. It has been replaced in many products by aspartame (NutraSweet). In 1997, the diet-food industry began pressuring the U.S. and Canadian governments and the World Health Organization to take saccharin off their lists of cancer-causing chemicals. The industry acknowledges that saccharin causes bladder cancer in male rats, but argues that those tumors are caused by a mechanism that would not occur in humans. Many public health experts respond by stating that, even if that still-unproved mechanism were correct in male rats, saccharin could cause cancer by additional mechanisms and that, in some studies, saccharin has caused bladder cancer in mice and in female rats and other cancers in both rats and mice.

✂ SALATRIM . . .
Modified fat:
Baked goods,
candy.

This manufactured fat (developed by Nabisco) has the physical properties of regular fat, but the manufacturer claims it provides only about 5/9 as many calories. Its use can enable companies to make reduced-calorie claims on their products. Salatrim's low calorie content results from its content of stearic acid, which the manufacturer says is absorbed poorly, and short-chain fatty acids, which provide fewer calories per unit weight.

Critics have charged that it does not provide as big a calorie reduction as claimed by Nabisco. Moreover, only very limited testing has been done to determine effects on humans. Eating small amounts of salatrim is probably safe, but large amounts (30g or more per day) increase the risk of such side effects as stomach cramps and nausea. No tests have been done to determine if the various food additives (salatrim, olestra, mannitol, and sorbitol) that cause gastrointestinal symptoms can act in concert to cause greater effects.

Nabisco declared salatrim safe and has marketed it, as the law allows, without formal FDA approval. (Nabisco has since sold salatrim to another company, Cultor.) In June 1998, the Center for Science in the Public Interest urged the FDA to ban salatrim until better tests were done and demonstrated safety.

✂ SALT (Sodium
Chloride) . . .
Flavoring: Most
processed foods,
soup, potato
chips, crackers.

Salt is used liberally in many processed foods and restaurant meals. Other additives contribute additional sodium. A diet high in sodium increases the risk or severity of high blood pressure, which increases the risk of heart attack and stroke. Everyone should eat less salt: avoid salty processed foods and restaurant meals, use salt sparingly, and enjoy other seasonings.

✓ SODIUM BENZOATE
. . . Preservative:
Fruit juice,

Manufacturers have used sodium benzoate for a century to prevent the growth of microorganisms in acidic foods.

carbonated drinks,
pickles, preserves.

✓ SODIUM CARBOXY-
METHYLCELLULOSE
(CMC) . . .
Thickening and
stabilizing agent;
prevents sugar
from crystallizing:
Ice cream, beer,
pie fillings, icings,
diet foods, candy.

CMC is made by reacting cellulose with a
derivative of acetic acid. Studies indicate it
is safe.

⊘ SODIUM NITRITE,
SODIUM NITRATE
. . . Preservative,
coloring, flavoring:
Bacon, ham,
frankfurters,
luncheon meats,
smoked fish,
corned beef.

Meat processors love sodium nitrite because
it stabilizes the red color in cured meat
(without nitrite, hot dogs and bacon would
look gray) and gives a characteristic flavor.
Sodium nitrate is used in dry cured meat,
because it slowly breaks down into nitrite.
Adding nitrite to food can lead to the
formation of small amounts of potent
cancer-causing chemicals (nitrosamines),
particularly in fried bacon. Nitrite, which
also occurs in saliva and forms from nitrate
in several vegetables, can undergo the same
chemical reaction in the stomach.
Companies now add ascorbic acid or erythorbic acid to bacon to inhibit nitrosamine
formation, a measure that has greatly
reduced the problem. While nitrite and
nitrate cause only a small risk, they are still
worth avoiding.

Several studies have linked consumption
of cured meat and nitrite by children, pregnant women, and adults with various types
of cancer. Although those studies have not
yet proven that eating nitrite in bacon,
sausage, and ham causes cancer in humans,
pregnant women would be prudent to
avoid those products.

The meat industry justifies its use of
nitrite and nitrate by claiming that it prevents the growth of bacteria that cause botulism poisoning. That's true, but freezing
and refrigeration could also do that, and the

U.S. Department of Agriculture has developed a safe method using lactic-acid-producing bacteria. The use of nitrite and nitrate has decreased greatly over the decades, because of refrigeration and restrictions on the amounts used. The meat industry could do the public's health a favor by cutting back even further. Because nitrite is used primarily in fatty, salty foods, consumers have important nutritional reasons for avoiding nitrite-preserved foods.

✓ SORBIC ACID, POTASSIUM SORBATE . . . Prevents growth of mold: Cheese, syrup, jelly, cake, wine, dry fruits.

Sorbic acid occurs naturally in many plants. These additives are safe.

✓ SORBITAN MONOSTEARATE . . . Emulsifier: Cakes, candy, frozen pudding, icing.

Like mono- and diglycerides and polysorbates, this additive keeps oil and water mixed together. In chocolate candy, it prevents the discoloration that normally occurs when the candy is warmed up and then cooled down.

✂ SORBITOL . . . Sweetener, thickening agent, maintains moisture. Dietetic drinks and foods, candy, shredded coconut, chewing gum.

Sorbitol occurs naturally in fruits and berries and is a close relative of sugars. It is half as sweet as sugar. It is used in many dietetic foods. It is used in non-cariogenic (non-decay-causing) chewing gum because oral bacteria do not metabolize it well. Some diabetics use sorbitol-sweetened foods because it is absorbed slowly and does not cause blood sugar to increase rapidly. Moderate amounts of sorbitol may have a strong laxative effect and even cause diarrhea, but otherwise it is safe.

✓ STARCH . . . Thickening agent: Soup, gravy.

Starch, the major component of flour, potatoes, and corn, is used in many foods as a thickening agent. However, starch does not dissolve in cold water. Chemists have solved this problem by reacting starch with various chemicals to create MODIFIED STARCHES (see next entry).

✓ STARCH, MODIFIED ... Thickening agent: Soup, gravy, baby food.

Modified starches are used in processed foods to improve their consistency and keep the solids suspended. Starch and modified starches sometimes replace large percentages of more nutritious ingredients, such as fruit. Choose baby foods without added starches (starch-thickened baby foods have contained as little as 25 percent as much of the fruit ingredients as 100-percent-fruit baby foods). One small study suggested that modified starches can promote diarrhea in infants.

✓ SUCRALOSE ... Artificial sweetener: Diet foods.

Approved in the United States in April 1998, sucralose (a synthetic chemical) can be used in soft drinks, baked goods, ice cream, sweetener packets, and other products. It previously had been used in Canada, Europe, and elsewhere. Sucralose is safer than saccharin and cyclamate and doesn't raise the concerns that tests on acesulfame-K and aspartame have raised.

✂ SUGAR (SUCROSE) ... Sweetener: Table sugar, sweetened foods.

Sucrose, ordinary table sugar, occurs naturally in fruit, sugar cane, and sugar beets. Americans consume about 65 pounds of sucrose per year. That figure is down from 102 pounds per year around 1970, but the decrease has been more than made up for with HIGH-FRUCTOSE CORN SYRUP and DEXTROSE. About 156 pounds of all refined sugars are produced per person per year, an increase of 28 percent since 1983. Interestingly that's just when the use of ASPARTAME started skyrocketing. In other words, it appears that artificial sweeteners have not replaced sugar, but may have stimulated America's sweet tooth.

Sugar and sweetened foods may taste good and supply energy, but most people eat too much of them. Sugar, corn syrup, and other refined sweeteners make up 16 percent of the average diet, but provide no vitamins, minerals, or protein. That means that a person would have to get 100 percent of his or her nutrients from only 84 percent of his or her food. Sugar and other refined sugars can promote obesity, tooth decay, and, in people with high triglycerides, heart disease.

▲ SULFITES (SULFUR DIOXIDE, SODIUM BISULFITE) . . . Preservative, bleach: Dried fruit, wine, processed potatoes.

Sulfiting agents prevent discoloration (dried fruit, some "fresh" shrimp, and some dried, fried, or frozen potatoes) and bacterial growth (wine). They also destroy vitamin B-1 and, most important, can cause severe reactions, especially in asthmatics. If you think you may be sensitive, avoid all forms of this additive, because it has caused at least twelve known deaths and probably many more.

✓ THIAMIN MONO-NITRATE . . . Vitamin B-1.

Perfectly safe, despite adding minuscule amounts of nitrate to our food.

✓ VANILLIN, ETHYL VANILLIN . . . Substitute for vanilla: Ice cream, baked goods, beverages, chocolate, candy, gelatin desserts.

Vanilla flavoring is derived from a bean, but vanillin, the major flavor component of vanilla, is cheaper to produce in a factory. A derivative, ethyl vanillin, comes closer to matching the taste of real vanilla. Both chemicals are safe.

✓ VEGETABLE OIL STEROLS . . . Cholesterol-lowering Additive: Margarine, other foods.

These substances, which are extracted from soybeans, reduce the absorption of cholesterol from food and lower blood-cholesterol levels. They are not toxic, but they may reduce the body's absorption of nutrients called carotenoids that are thought to reduce the risk of cancer and heart disease. Used in Take Control–brand margarine.

The food and chemical industries have said for decades that all food additives are well tested and safe. And most additives are safe. However, the history of food additives is riddled with additives that, after many years of use, were found to pose health risks. Those listed below have been banned. The moral of the story is that when someone says that all food additives are well tested and safe you should take their assurances with a grain of salt.

Food Additive Cemetery—Additives That Have Been Banned

Additive	Function	Natural or Synthetic	Year Banned	Problem
Agene (nitrogen trichloride)	flour bleaching and aging agent	synthetic	1949	dogs that ate bread made from treated flour suffered epileptic-like fits; the toxic agent was methionine sulfoxime
• Butter yellow	artificial coloring	synthetic	1919	toxic, later found to cause liver cancer
• Green 1	artificial coloring	synthetic	1965	liver cancer
• Green 2	artificial coloring	synthetic	1965	insufficient economic importance to be tested
• Orange 1	artificial coloring	synthetic	1956	organ damage
• Orange 2	artificial coloring	synthetic	1960	organ damage
• Orange B	artificial coloring	synthetic	1978 (ban never finalized)	cancer
• Red 1	artificial coloring	synthetic	1961	liver cancer
• Red 2	artificial coloring	synthetic	1976	possible carcinogen
• Red 4	artificial coloring	synthetic	1976	high levels damaged adrenal cortex of dog; after 1965 it was used only in maraschino cherries and certain pills; it is still allowed in externally applied drugs and cosmetics
• Red 32	artificial coloring	synthetic	1956	damages internal organs and may be a weak carcinogen; since 1956 it continues to be used under the name Citrus Red 2 only to color oranges (2 ppm)
• Sudan 1	artificial coloring	synthetic	1919	toxic, later found to be carcinogenic

Additive	Function	Natural or Synthetic	Year Banned	Problem
• Violet 1	artificial coloring	synthetic	1973	cancer (it had been used to stamp the Department of Agriculture's inspection mark on beef carcasses)
• Yellow 1 and 2	artificial coloring	synthetic	1959	intestinal lesions at high dosages
• Yellow 3	artificial coloring	synthetic	1959	heart damage at high dosages
• Yellow 4	artificial coloring	synthetic	1959	heart damage at high dosages
cinnamyl anthranilate	artificial flavoring	synthetic	1982	liver cancer
cobalt salts	stabilize beer foam	synthetic	1966	toxic effects on heart
coumarin	flavoring	tonka bean	1954	liver poison
cyclamate	artificial sweetener	synthetic	1970	bladder cancer, damage to testes; now not thought to cause cancer directly, but to increase the potency of other carcinogens
diethyl pyrocarbonate (DEPC)	preservative (beverages)	synthetic	1972	combines with ammonia to form urethane, a carcinogen
dulcin (p-ethoxy-phenylurea)	artificial sweetener	synthetic	1950	liver cancer
ethylene glycol	solvent	humectant	synthetic	kidney damage
monochloroacetic acid	preservative	synthetic	1941	highly toxic
nordihydroguaiaretic adic (NDGA)	antioxidant	desert plant	1968 (FDA) 1971 (USDA)	kidney damage
oil of calamus	flavoring	root of calamus	1968	intestinal cancer
polyoxyethylene-8-stearate (Myrj 45)	emulsifier	synthetic	1952	high levels caused bladder stones and tumors
safrole	flavoring (root beer)	sassafras	1960	liver cancer
thiourea	preservative	synthetic	c. 1950	liver cancer

5

Directory of Organizations

Many organizations around the world are working to improve food safety at local, national, and international levels. Most local, regional, and national governments have agencies that specifically promote food safety by making and enforcing laws and regulations. Nonprofit organizations worldwide are committed to food safety improvements, although they don't always agree about how they should be accomplished. For some of the organizations listed here, food safety is their primary focus. For others, food safety fits in with their general focus on consumer, humanitarian, or environmental issues. Besides the organizations listed here, there are many trade organizations established to promote a particular foodstuff that also have food safety programs. Most of these organizations have websites that can be found by entering the name of the foodstuff and the word "board" or "commission" in a search engine (for example, "egg board").

Nonprofit, Trade, and Professional Organizations

Alliance for Bio-Integrity
406 W. Depot Avenue
Fairfield, IA 52556
Phone: (515) 472-5554
Fax: (515) 472-6431
Website: http://www.biointegrity.org

The Alliance for Bio-Integrity is a nonprofit, nonpolitical organization working to advance human and environmental health through sustainable and safe technologies. The organization is a coalition of both scientists and religious leaders who believe that genetically engineered food is harmful to the environment and contrary to many religious beliefs. The alliance has filed suit against the FDA to require genetically altered food to undergo the same testing procedures as new food additives and to require genetically altered foods to be labeled for consumers.

Information about the lawsuit and statements by scientists about genetically engineered food are included at the website.

American Council on Science and Health
1995 Broadway
Second Floor
New York, NY 10023
Phone: (212) 362-7044
Fax: (212) 362-4919
Website: http://www.acsh.org

The American Council on Science and Health is funded by pesticide manufacturers, food companies, pharmaceutical companies, and trade associations to provide information to consumers about food, nutrition, chemicals, pharmaceuticals, lifestyle, the environment, and health. The council publishes a wide variety of pamphlets and reports on food, health, and environmental topics.

All of the council's publications are available for download at the website.

American Dietetic Association
216 W. Jackson Boulevard
Chicago, IL 60606
Phone: (312) 899-0040
Website: www.eatright.org

The American Dietetic Association is the primary professional organization of U.S. dietitians. Although the emphasis is nutrition in general, food safety is an area of interest. The association publishes *The Journal of the American Dietetic Association*.

The website is quite extensive. There are many nutrition fact sheets available including some on food safety.

American Public Health Association (APHA)
800 I Street NW
Washington, DC 20001
Phone: (202) 777-2742
Fax: (202) 777-2532
Website: http://www.apha.org

The American Public Health Association has over fifty thousand members in over fifty occupations in public health. APHA helps set public health standards, works with national and international health agencies to improve health worldwide, and provides public health professionals with resources for professional exchange, study, and action. Two of their practice sections have particular application to food safety: the Food and Nutrition Section contributes to long-range planning in food, nutrition, and health policy, and the Epidemiology Section works to disseminate new scientific information to improve development, implementation, and evaluation of policies impacting public health.

Program information and links to other epidemiology websites are included on this website.

Aspartame Consumer Safety Network and Pilots Hotline
P.O. Box 780634
Dallas, TX 75378
Phone: (214) 352-4268
Website: http://web2airmail.net/marystod/

The Aspartame Consumer Safety Network and Pilots Hotline supports people who have had adverse reactions to aspartame (marketed under the names NutraSweet and Equal) with information and legislative efforts to restrict the substance. Aspartame generates more complaints to the FDA from consumers than any other food additive.

The website has a questionnaire to determine aspartame sensitivity, information about aspartame, and the activities of the organization.

Association of Food and Drug Officials (AFDO)
P.O. Box 3425
2250 Kingston Road, Suite 311
York, PA 17402
Phone: (717) 757-2888

Fax: (717) 755-8089
Website: http://www.afdo.org

Association of Food and Drug Officials (AFDO) is an international organization devoted to developing strategies to promote public health and resolve consumer protection issues related to the regulation of foods, drugs, medical devices, and consumer products. AFDO promotes uniform and rational regulation. Members include local, state, and federal regulators, as well as representatives from academia and industry.

Position statements, HACCP training programs, and program information are provided on the website.

Center for Food Safety (CFS)
International Center for Technology Assessment
310 D Street NE
Washington, DC 20002
Phone: (202) 547-9359
Fax: (202) 547-9429
E-mail: office@icta.org
Website: http://www.icta.org

The Center for Food Safety (CFS) is a project of the International Center for Technology Assessment that works to ensure that technology is used in responsible ways. The goals of CFS include promoting sustainable, organic agricultural practices and ensuring testing and labeling of genetically engineered food. They use grassroots campaigns, media outreach, public education, and litigation to advance their goals. Two of their projects, Organic Watch, a group of organizations, and Organic Food Action Network, a consumer group, work to maintain the integrity of the organic food standard.

Center for Science in the Public Interest (CSPI)
1875 Connecticut Avenue NW, Suite 300
Washington, DC 20009
Phone: (202) 332-9110
Fax: (202) 265-4954
E-mail: cspi@cspinet.org
Website: http://cspinet.org

The Center for Science in the Public Interest (CSPI) is a nonprofit education and advocacy organization that works to improve the safety and nutritional quality of our food supply. Reducing damage that results from consuming alcoholic beverages is another important aspect of their work. Some of their recent projects include working to reduce antibiotic use in animals, calling for stronger international food safety rules, monitoring new additives, and working to reduce soda consumption in children. CSPI has more than 1 million members and produces the outstanding *Nutrition Action Letter*, which keeps its members abreast of food safety and nutrition issues.

Their website provides information about campaigns, food additives, food safety, and current projects.

Community Nutrition Institute (CNI)
910 17th Street NW, Suite 800
Washington, DC 20006
Phone: (202) 776-0595
Fax: (202) 776-0599

Community Nutrition Institute was founded in 1970 to promote consumer protection, food program development and management, and sound federal diet and health policies. CNI developed the legislative basis for the Women, Infants, and Children (WIC) nutrition program and successfully lobbied Congress for funding the WIC program. Currently CNI monitors nutrition labeling, meat and poultry inspection, hunger programs, and the use of chemicals in the U.S. food supply. CNI has sued federal agencies to maintain quality food standards; has testified before congressional, state legislative, and executive branch committees; and is a source of expertise and comment on food issues to the media.

Consumer's Union
1666 Connecticut Avenue NW, Suite 310
Washington, DC 20009-1039
Phone: (202) 462-6262
Fax: (202) 265-9548
Website: www.consumersunion.org

Since its founding in 1936, Consumer's Union has been a highly regarded nonprofit testing and information organization, serving consumers only. Its mission is to test products, inform the public, and protect consumers. It publishes *Consumer Reports*, testifies on behalf of consumers before state and federal legislative and regulatory bodies, petitions government agencies, and files lawsuits on behalf of the consumer interest.

A variety of articles and position papers from technical reports to articles that have appeared in *Consumer Reports* are available at the website.

Dairy Food Safety Laboratory (DFSL)
Veterinary Medicine Teaching and Research Center
18830 Road 112
Tulare, CA 93274
Phone: (559) 688-1731
Website: www.vetmed.ucdavis.edu/dfsl/dfs/main.html

The Dairy Food Safety Laboratory was established in 1992 by the University of California at Davis and the Veterinary Medicine Teaching and Research Center to perform rapid-response, applied research on herd health and on food safety problems that originate on farms. The DFSL provides educational opportunities for students from high school through postdoctoral fellows, gives talks to consumers, producers, veterinarians, regulators, and students, and publishes its research findings in scientific journals.

Environmental Working Group (EWG)
1718 Connecticut Avenue NW, Suite 600
Washington, DC 20009
Phone: (202) 667-6982
Fax: (202) 232-2592
http://www.ewg.org
Website: http://www.ewg.org

Since its founding in 1993, the Environmental Working Group has produced reports and articles, and given technical assistance to over four hundred public interest groups. The EWG analyzes government and other data to produce hundreds of reports each year, many of which make headlines. Although the EWG works on a variety of environmental projects, pesticide use is an area of special emphasis, particularly when its use threatens the health of infants and children.

One interesting section of its very informative website is "Food News." This section has information on pesticides, including an interactive portion that calculates the level of pesticide residues in the user's diet. Other sections feature information about campaign contributions, reports, and other environmental issues.

Factory Farm Project
Global Resource Action Center for the Environment (GRACE)
15 E. 26th Street, Suite 915
New York, NY 10010
Phone: (212) 726-9161
Fax: (212) 726-9160
Website: http://www.factoryfarm.org

Established in 1996, GRACE works with research, policy, and grassroots organizations to preserve the future of the planet and protect the quality of the environment. One of GRACE's main projects is the Factory Farm Project, which works to eliminate factory farms as a mode of production, replacing them with sustainable food production systems that are healthful, economically viable, environmentally sound, and humane. Factory farming is a concern to many organizations, including animal rights groups, environmental protection groups, and food safety groups.

The website includes links to many organizations and articles regarding factory farms and links to various state agencies and organizations.

Food Allergy Network (FAN)
10400 Eaton Place, Suite 107
Fairfax, VA 22030
Phone: (800) 929-4040
Website: http://www.foodallergy.org

Food Allergy Network works to increase food allergy and anaphylaxis (a severe, life-threatening allergic reaction) awareness by contacts with media, education, publishing, advocacy, and research efforts. FAN can help allergic individuals with recipes, ingredients lists, strategies for dealing with allergies including negotiating restaurants, and techniques for administering life-saving drugs.

The website provides information about allergies, recipes, tips, research, and resources that can be ordered.

Food and Water
389 Vermont Route 215
Walden, VT 05873
Phone: (802) 563-3300
Fax: (802) 563-3310

Food and Water is a nonprofit advocacy organization that was founded by Walter Burnstein, a family physician who witnessed an extraordinary increase in degenerative diseases in his twenty-five years of practice. Food and Water's mission is to reduce the use of pesticides, hormones in animals, genetic engineering, and food irradiation. In addition to lobbying at the state and national levels, they publish the quarterly *Food and Water Journal*. (Yearly subscription rates are $25 for individuals, $40 for nonprofit organizations, and $100 for businesses.)

Food Animal Concerns Trust (FACT)
P.O. Box 14599
Chicago, IL 60614
Phone: (773) 525-4952
Website: http://www.fact.cc

Food Animal Concerns Trust (FACT) was established in 1982 to improve the welfare of farm animals; increase the safety of meat, milk, and eggs; broaden economic opportunities for family farmers; and reduce environmental pollution. FACT lobbies the Food and Drug Administration, the Department of Agriculture, and the Centers for Disease Control to implement regulations to reduce pathogens at the farm level. FACT also operates some demonstration farms to show how pathogens can be reduced and has recently begun a public education program.

Information about factory farming, foodborne illness, and programs appears on the website.

Food Research Institute
1925 Willow Drive
Madison, WI 53706
Phone: (608) 263-6955
E-mail: mwpariza@facstaff.wisc.edu
Website: http://www.foodsafety.org

The Food Research Institute is part of the University of Wisconsin–Madison. The institute works with industry regulators, academia, and consumers on food safety issues to provide accurate and useful information and expertise. The institute provides education and training in food safety, and the microbiology division conducts basic and applied research about food-associated illnesses caused by bacteria, molds, and viruses. Research is reported in journals; none of the research results are kept secret. At the consumer level, they are one of the sponsors of the National Food Safety Database.

Please see the database section for further information about this database.

Food Safety Consortium
110 Agricultural Building
University of Arkansas
Fayetteville, AR 72701
Phone: (501) 575-5647
Fax: (501) 575-7531
e-mail: fsc@cavern.uark.edu

The Food Safety Consortium is made up of researchers from the University of Arkansas, Iowa State University, and Kansas State University. It was established by the U.S. Congress in 1988 to conduct extensive food safety investigations into all areas of poultry, beef, and pork meat production, from the farm to the consumer's table. The consortium sponsors conferences and publishes food safety research.

Friends of the Earth (FOE)
1025 Vermont Avenue NW
Washington, DC 20005
Phone: (202) 783-7400
Fax: (202) 783-0444
E-mail: foe@foe.org
Website: http://www.foe.org

Friends of the Earth is a national environmental organization working to preserve the health and diversity of the planet for future generations. FOE is the largest international environmental network in the world with affiliates in sixty-three countries. FOE works on a variety of environmental issues. Its Safer Food, Safer Farms campaign seeks to reduce or eliminate the use of pesticides and eliminate genetically modified crops.

A well-organized website offers detailed information about the campaigns, fact sheets, links to other organizations, press releases, and sample letters to write.

Greenpeace USA
1436 U Street NW
Washington, DC 20009
Phone: (800) 326-0939
Website: http://www.greenpeaceusa.org

Greenpeace, a highly active environmental organization, opposes releasing genetically modified food into the environment. Specifically Greenpeace is lobbying governments to require segregation and labeling of genetically engineered foods so that consumers will be able to determine whether their foods have been genetically modified. Greenpeace has proposed labeling methods to the European Union. Another area of concern for Greenpeace is persistent organic pollutants (POPs). These substances get into food through the consumption of animal fats, pesticides, and packaging and processing material.

Policy statements and articles can be found on the website. For an international view, use the international website, http://www.greenpeace.org.

Institute of Food Science and Technology (IFST)
5 Cambridge Court
210 Shepherd's Bush Road
London, W6 7NJ United Kingdom
Website: http://www.ifst.org

Institute of Food Science and Technology (IFST) is an independent professional group of food scientists and technologists. The institute publishes position papers on a variety of food safety issues and promotes the application of science and technology to all aspects of the supply of safe, wholesome, nutritious, and attractive food.

Position papers as well as food safety FAQs are available at the website.

Institute of Food Technologists (IFT)
221 N. LaSalle Street, Suite 300
Chicago, IL 60601

Phone: (312) 782-8424
Fax: (312) 782-8348
Website: http://www.ift.org

The Institute of Food Technologists seeks to advance the science and technology of food through the exchange of knowledge and be recognized as an advocate for science on food-related issues. A professional organization for food technologists, the institute sponsors conferences, and provides an information gateway to over 2,200 food science and technology resources.

The institute has one of the best websites for food safety research. The food headlines section contains summaries of current food-related news stories, and an information gateway provides links to over two thousand websites on a variety of topics. Best of all, the websites featured represent all different points of view.

International Association for Food Protection
(formerly International Association of Milk, Food, and Environmental Sanitarians)
6200 Aurora Avenue, Suite 200 W
Des Moines, IA 50322
Phone: (800) 369-6337
Fax: (515) 276-8655
Website: http://www.foodprotection.org

The association works to keep its members, food safety professionals, informed of the latest scientific, technical, and practical developments in food safety and sanitation. The association produces two publications: *Dairy, Food, and Environmental Sanitation* is the membership magazine with articles on applied research and current applications of technology, and *The Journal of Food Protection* is a refereed journal of food microbiology.

Program information, current issue of *Dairy, Food, and Environmental Sanitation*, and index and abstracts of *Journal of Food Protection* are offered on the website.

International Commission on
Microbial Specifications for Food
International Union of Microbiological Societies
Chairman: T. A. Roberts

Consultant Food Safety
59 Edenham Crescent
Berkeley Avenue
Reading, RG1 6HV United Kingdom
Website: http://www.cairo.au/icmsf.htm

The International Commission on Microbial Specifications for Food is a nonprofit scientific advisory body established under the auspices of the International Union of Microbiological Societies to address food microbiological concerns. It has developed methods, sampling plans, microbiological criteria, and HACCP plans. Several books have been published in its series, Microorganisms in Food. It advises national governments as well as international bodies such as Codex Alimentarius, World Health Organization, and the International Atomic Energy Agency.

Program information and details about the Microorganisms in Food series may also be found on its website.

The International Food Information Council
1100 Connecticut Avenue NW, Suite 430
Washington, DC 20036
Phone: (202) 296-6540
E-mail: foodinfo@ific.health.org
Website: http://www.ificinfo.health.org

The International Food Information Council (IFIC) was founded in 1985 to provide information about food safety and nutrition to consumers. It is funded by food, beverage, and agricultural companies but does not represent any product or company and does not lobby for legislative or regulatory action. One of its recent educational efforts is about the Delaney amendment. IFIC argues that these amendments, which prevent cancer-causing agents in food, are too far-reaching and should be modified.

There is a lot of information about food safety issues from an industry point of view on its website.

International Food Safety Council
Education Foundation of the National Restaurant Association
1200 17th Street NW
Washington, DC 20036

Phone: (312) 715-5368
Website: www.foodsafetycouncil.org

A coalition of restaurant and food service professionals who are certified in safe food handling and preparation, the International Food Safety Council promotes food safety education within the food service industry and works to convey the industry's commitment to serve safe food to the public. As part of this commitment, the council sponsors National Food Safety Education Month each September. It is a founding sponsor of the Partnership for Food Safety Education and publishes *Best Practices*, an industry publication that features practical ways to enhance food safety in various operations.

The website provides program information, safe food handling in the home, and a food safety quiz.

Joint Institute for Food Safety and Applied Nutrition (JIFSAN)
University of Maryland
College Park, MD 20742
Phone: (301) 405-8382
Website: http://www.jifsan.umd.edu

The Joint Institute for Food Safety and Applied Nutrition was established as a joint project of USFDA and the University of Maryland in 1996 to be a multidisciplinary research and education program to provide a scientific basis for ensuring a safe, wholesome food supply. The program includes an academic and regulatory sciences program, policy studies, and outreach and education programs. Recent research programs include risk analysis, microbial pathogens and toxins, food composition and applied nutrition, and animal health sciences as they affect food safety.

The website includes a program description and information on meetings, workshops, grants, education, and outreach programs.

Lois Joy Galler Foundation for Hemolytic Uremic Syndrome
734 Walt Whitman Road
Melville, NY 11747
Phone: (516) 673-3017

Fax: (516) 673-3025
Website: http://www.loisjoygaller.org

The Lois Joy Galler Foundation for Hemolytic Uremic Syndrome was established by Lois Joy Galler's parents after she died of hemolytic uremic syndrome (HUS), a complication that can develop after infection with *E. coli* O157:H7. The foundation was established to raise money for research on HUS to prevent and cure the disease. Raising public awareness and providing a supportive community for the families of affected children are other goals of the organization. One of the ways they provide support is by maintaining a list of parents that are willing to talk to others who have been affected. They have also produced a videotape about the syndrome.

Program information and facts about HUS appear on the website.

Mothers & Others
40 West 20th Street
New York, NY 10011
Phone: (212) 242-0010
Website: www.mothers.org

Mothers & Others was founded in 1989 by actress Meryl Streep and her Connecticut neighbors because of concern that children were being exposed to unsafe levels of pesticides from food. Since mothers are often their family's principal shopper, the organization was established to harness consumer power toward safer, ecologically sustainable food sources. The organization has been remarkably effective at raising awareness for children's exposure to pesticides. In 1997 the U.S. Environmental Protection Agency announced its National Agenda to Protect Children from Environmental Threats and has since set reduced pesticide tolerance levels based on computations for children.

The website offers resources for shoppers who want to support organic and hormone-free foods as well as political action opportunities to influence government and corporations to make food safer.

Mothers for Natural Law
P.O. Box 1177
Fairfield, IA 52556

Phone: (515) 472-2809
Fax: (515) 472-2683
E-mail: mothers@safe-food.org
Website: http://www.safe-food.org

Mothers for Natural Law is a consumer group concerned with the proliferation of genetically engineered food. They are coordinating a right-to-know campaign to secure laws that would ensure rigorous, premarket testing and mandatory labeling of genetically engineered food. They also serve as a resource for consumers, food manufacturers, and food processors looking for sources of genetically natural foods.

In addition to information about genetically engineered crops and their political campaigns, the website has a database of nongenetically engineered foods.

National Center for Food Safety and Technology (NCFST)
6502 S. Archer Road
Summit-Argo, IL 60501
Phone: (708) 563-1576
Fax: (708) 563-1873
Website: http://www.iit.edu/~ncfs/

National Center for Food Safety and Technology is a consortium of food companies, the U.S. Food and Drug Administration, and university-based scientists working together to ensure the safety of food processing and packaging technologies. This objective is met through a combination of research and outreach within the food science community. Research areas include finding scientific bases to answer regulatory questions related to food safety and conducting research to promote the safety and quality of the U.S. food supply. Outreach activities include publications in journals, presentations, workshops, training programs, degree and certificate programs, tours, and consultation services.

The website has program information.

National Environmental Health Association
700 S. Colorado Boulevard
South Tower, Suite 970
Denver, CO 80246
Phone: (303) 756-9090

Fax: (303) 691-9490
Website: http://www.neha.org

A national professional society for environmental health practitioners, the National Environmental Health Association offers eight credential programs including Certified Food Safety Professional. The certification requires a combination of education, experience, and passage of an exam. The association publishes the *Journal of Environmental Health* and *Food and Environment News Digest*.

In addition to program information, position papers on various food safety issues are available on the website.

National Organization Mobilized to Stop Glutamate (NoMSG)
P.O. Box 367
Santa Fe, NM 87504
Phone: (800) 232-8674
Fax: (505) 424-0444
Website: http://www.nomsg.com

National Organization Mobilized to Stop Glutamate (NoMSG) estimates that one-quarter of the world's population reacts negatively to monosodium glutamate (MSG). NoMSG works to educate consumers regarding the dangers of MSG and the ways it can be hidden, encourage MSG-free products, support MSG-sensitive individuals, and support research.

The website provides information about lobby groups, hidden sources of MSG, common reactions, books about MSG, and a discussion board.

National Restaurant Association
1200 17th Street NW
Washington, DC 20036
Phone: (800) 424-5156
Fax: (202) 331-2429
Website: http://www.restaurant.org

The National Restaurant Association was established in 1923 to educate and represent its members and to promote the restaurant industry. Although they have many activities, food safety is a priority. Their education foundation created the *ServSafe* food safety training course in the 1970s. The program is recognized and accepted by more federal, state, and local jurisdictions than any other food safety education and training program.

The website provides program information, training materials, and links to Food Safety Information Council.

Natural Resources Defense Council (NRDC)
40 W. 20th Street
New York, NY 10011
Phone: (212) 727-2700
Website: http://www.nrdc.org

The Natural Resources Defense Council (NRDC) uses law, science, and the efforts of its more than 400,000 members to protect wildlife, open spaces, and ensure a safe and healthy environment for all living things. NRDC produced a study in 1989 documenting the dangers of the pesticide Alar called "Intolerable Risk: Pesticides in Our Children's Food." The study was publicized on *60 Minutes* and caused the withdrawal of Alar from the U.S. market. NRDC has continued to lobby against dangerous pesticides and supports organic farming methods and pesticide reduction.

Detailed reports as well as links to other organizations are available at this website.

NSF International
P.O. Box 130140
789 N. Dixboro Road
Ann Arbor, MI 48113
Phone: (800) NSF-MARK
Fax: (734) 769-0109
Website: http://www.nsf.org

NSF International, formerly known as the National Sanitation Foundation, was founded in 1944 as an independent nonprofit organization to develop sanitation standards, provide education, and perform third-party conformity audits. One of its largest programs is the NSF certification program. Manufacturers can submit their products to NSF for testing. If the product meets NSF standards, the NSF mark is placed on the product. NSF enforces the standards of the mark and will take legal action against companies if the products later fail to meet NSF standards.

The website offers information on program services, standards, and accreditation.

Organic Consumers Association
860 Highway 61
Little Marais, MN 55614
Phone: (218) 226-4164
Fax: (218) 226-4157
E-mail: alliance@mr.net
Website: http://www.purefood.org

Formerly known as the Pure Food Campaign, Organic Consumers Association works to promote organic and sustainable farming worldwide. Areas of particular concern for the organization are genetically engineered food, bovine growth hormone, irradiation, and cloning. The campaign uses public education, targeted boycotts, grassroots lobbying, litigation, activist networking, direct action protests, and media events. They also produce two electronic newsletters: *Campaign for Food Safety News* and *Organic Views*.

In addition to a lot of information about a variety of food safety issues, a database of health food stores and suppliers is available on the website.

Partnership for Food Safety Education
800 Connecticut Avenue NW, Suite 500
Washington, DC 20006-2701
Phone: (202) 429-8273
Website: http://www.fightbac.org

The Partnership for Food Safety Education was created in 1997 as a coalition of ten industry, consumer, and government agencies concerned about food safety and now has twenty-one organizational members. The partnership has created an educational campaign to teach children, the general public, and people who are at high risk for foodborne illness about ways to improve food safety. The campaign—called Fight BAC!—is divided into four elements: cook, clean, separate, and chill. Each message is age appropriate. For example, preschoolers are encouraged to wash their hands and rinse fruits and vegetables. Campaigns aimed at adults have featured proper ways to grill meats, and campaigns for restaurant workers stress proper sanitation.

The website features food safety information and ordering information for teaching materials.

Pesticide Action Network
North American Regional Center
49 Powell Street, Suite 50
San Francisco, CA 94102
Phone: (415) 981-1771
Fax: (415) 981-1991
E-mail: panna@panna.org
Website: http://www.panna.org

The Pesticide Action Network works to replace pesticides with ecologically sound alternatives worldwide. The North American branch (PANNA) was founded in 1982 to link over 130 affiliated health, consumer, labor, environment, progressive agriculture, and public interest groups in Canada, the United States, and Mexico with more than 400 partners worldwide to promote healthier, more effective pest management. The network uses education, media, demonstration projects, and international advocacy campaigns to promote pesticide alternatives. *Global Pesticide Campaign* is produced quarterly ($25 for individuals, $50 for libraries, and $100 for corporations) and contains articles on pesticides and sustainable agriculture, health, labor, food security, environmental issues, pesticide manufacturers, and politics.

The website has some issues of *Global Pesticide Campaign*, and the Pesticide Information Service database (*PESTIS*) containing pesticide reform–related materials, including articles, newsletters, reports, and action alerts not just from PANNA but from other related organizations as well.

Physicians for Social Responsibility
Environment and Health Program
1101 14th Street NW, Suite 700
Washington, DC 20005
Phone: (202) 898-0150
Fax: (202) 898-0172
Website: http://www.psr.org

The Environment and Health Program of Physicians for Social Responsibility (PSR) is designed to address the challenges to human health posed by contamination of the environment due to human activities. The program is concerned with pesticides and safe food and water as well as clean air and children's environmental health. PSR serves as secretariat for the International Persistent Organic Pollutants Elimination Network (IPEN), a coalition of organizations working to eliminate carbon-based chemical compounds (like PCBs, pesticides, and dioxin) from industrial chemicals. These substances accumulate in the fatty tissues of living organisms and have been documented to cause many health problems for species at the top of the food chain, including predator animals and humans. Humans consume them by eating animal fats, pesticide residues, and foods that are contaminated from contact with packaging materials or bleached paper products such as coffee filters.

Information and links to IPEN are available at the website.

Public Citizen
1600 20th Street NW
Washington, DC 20009
Phone: (800) 289-3787
Website: www.citizen.org

Ralph Nader founded Public Citizen in 1971 to be the consumer's eyes and ears in Washington. Public Citizen has broad interests; however, two of its areas of concern are food safety and food irradiation.

The website offers program information and links to organizations and articles about irradiation and food safety.

Safe Food Coalition
888 17th Street NW, #800
Washington, DC 20006
Phone: (202) 822-8060
Fax: (202) 822-9088
E-mail: Cgould@fhminc.com

The Safe Food Coalition is a group of consumer, public health, whistleblower, senior citizen, and labor organizations that work together to promote food safety. Before the coalition takes a position on an issue, a position statement is circulated among the members, and any disagreements are negotiated. The coalition works to educate the public about the hazards of foodborne illness and testifies before Congress and government agencies to improve meat, poultry, and seafood inspections.

Safe Food for the Hungry

Purdue University's School of Consumer and Family Sciences
1260 Stone Hall
West Lafayette, IN 47907
Phone: (765) 494-8213
Website: http://www.cfs.purdue.edu/safefood/sfhungry.html

The goal of the program is to ensure safe food in soup kitchens and food distribution centers for the poor and to enable poor people to eat safely at home or wherever they consume food. Primarily an information organization, they publish a lot of nutrition education material, including nutritional needs through the life cycle. The most innovative materials show how to modify the food pyramid for foods that don't require cooking or refrigeration, and how to modify the pyramid for people of different cultural backgrounds who favor foods other than those in the typical American diet.

Lots of nutrition and program information is available on its website.

Safe Tables Our Priority (STOP)

335 Court Street, Suite 100
Brooklyn, NY 11231
General information: (718) 246-2739
Victims and families: (800) 350-STOP
E-mail: feedback@stop-usa.org
Website: http://www.stop-usa.org

Safe Tables Our Priority (STOP) was founded in 1993 as a support organization for victims of foodborne illnesses and their families. It has three main goals: (1) provision of information and services to those made ill by food, (2) prevention of foodborne illnesses through consumer education, and (3) reform of government and industry practices that allow pathogenic contamination of food. STOP is credited by the United States Department of Agriculture (USDA) and President Clinton as being instrumental in effecting the first meat and poultry reform in over ninety years. New regulations require science-based government inspections including tests for salmonella and require companies to conduct microbial testing for bacteria. STOP is a member of the Safe Food Coalition.

This website includes information for victims about illnesses and treatment options, food safety facts, status of pertinent legislation, and links to other organizations.

Society for Nutrition Education
1001 Connecticut Avenue NW, Suite 528
Washington, DC 20036
Phone: (202) 452-8534
Fax: (202) 452-8536
Website: http://www.sne.org

A professional society, Society for Nutrition Education (SNE) is dedicated to promoting healthy, sustainable food choices. Its members, nutrition educators, educate individuals, families, fellow professionals, and students and influence policymakers about nutrition, food, and health. The organization publishes the *Journal of Nutrition Education.*

Program and contact information is provided on the website.

Truth in Labeling Campaign
P.O. Box 2532
Darien, IL 60561
Phone: (858) 481-9333
Website: http://www.truthinlabeling.org

The Truth in Labeling Campaign is a nonprofit organization working to have all food containing monosodium glutamate (MSG) clearly labeled. Currently MSG can be included in such ingredients as yeast extract and natural flavoring without separate labeling. Since 1997, the Environmental Protection Agency (EPA) has approved MSG for spraying on crops. MSG is a neurotoxin that affects some people with migraine headaches, asthma, nausea and vomiting, fatigue, disorientation, and depression.

The website contains information about lobbying efforts, how MSG is hidden in food ingredients, and how to determine whether you're sensitive to MSG.

Union of Concerned Scientists
2 Brattle Square
Cambridge, MA 02238-9105

Phone: (617) 547-5552
Fax: (617) 864-9405
E-mail: ucs@ucsusa.org
Website: http://www.ucsusa.org

The Union of Concerned Scientists is a nonprofit organization that works to advance responsible public policy regarding technology. UCS advocates sustainable agriculture policies and practices to reduce agriculture's impact on the environment and to ensure economic stability and food security. Its main goals include promoting agricultural practices that minimize pesticide, fertilizer, and energy use and researching and evaluating the risks and benefits of biotechnology in agriculture. The union publishes *The Gene Exchange*, a newsletter about current developments in biotechnology, several times per year. It is available by e-mail or regular mail. UCS also publish *Nucleus*, which includes information on its research findings and progress reports on policy work as well as updates on legislative decisions in a variety of areas.

Information about the union's activities and articles from *The Gene Exchange* are available on the website.

National Agencies

Canada

Canadian Food Inspection Agency
Agriculture and Agri-Food Canada
59 Camelot Drive
Nepean, Ontario K1A OY9
Phone: (613) 952-8000

Canada recently consolidated several agencies to create the Canadian Food Inspection Agency. It is responsible for inspection services related to food safety as well as animal and plant health programs.

Division of Foodborne and Enteric Disease
Environmental Health Directorate
Health Canada
Environmental Health Center, Building #8
Tunney's Pasture

Ottawa, Ontario K1A O12
Phone: (613) 957-4243
Fax: (613) 941-7708

The Division of Foodborne and Enteric Disease works to assess and reduce the risk of foodborne, waterborne, and enteric disease in Canadians through national surveillance and targeted special studies.

Food Directorate
Health Protection Branch
Health Canada
Tunney's Pasture
Ottawa, Ontario K1A O12
Phone: (613) 967-1821
Fax: (613) 957-1784

The Food Directorate is responsible for food safety policy, standard setting, risk assessment, analytic research, and auditing food safety records.

United States

Center for Food Safety and Applied Nutrition
United States Food and Drug Administration
5600 Fishers Lane
Rockville, MD 20857
Phone: (800) 332-4010
Website: http://www.vm.cfsan.fda.gov/~lrd/cfsan2.html

The Center for Food Safety and Applied Nutrition is responsible for regulating $240 billion of domestic food as well as $15 billion of imported food. Regulations have the goal of ensuring that food is safe, nutritious, and wholesome, and that foods are honestly, accurately, and informatively labeled. In practice the FDA must approve all new foods, food additives, and drugs before they can be sold. Recently the center revamped food labels to make it easier for consumers to get nutrition information; approved certain health claims supported by scientific evidence showing a link between a food or nutrient and a disease or health condition (this allows manufacturers to advertise or label foods as having particular proven health benefits); and established new seafood regulations based on HACCP. FDA field personnel inspect food and cosmetics companies, examine food shipments from abroad, and collect samples that are tested in FDA labs. Compliance officers recommend legal action where appropriate and follow through with enforcement issues. The center also works with the Centers for Disease Control and Prevention and state health departments to resolve food safety concerns, and it works with Codex Alimentarius to help establish international food safety standards.

The website provides information about agency programs and links to related agencies.

Food Safety and Inspection Service
United States Department of Agriculture
Washington, DC 20250-3700
Phone: (202) 720-7943; Meat and poultry hotline: (800) 535-4555
Fax: (202) 720-1843
Website: http://www.fsis.usda.gov

The Food Safety and Inspection Service (FSIS), a branch of the USDA, is charged with ensuring the safety of all meat and poultry products sold in interstate and foreign commerce, including imported products. The FSIS uses 7,400 inspectors in 6,200 plants to check animals before and after slaughter, and performs microbiological tests to ensure that products meet safety standards.

FSIS sets standards for all aspects of meat processing, including evaluating food ingredients, additives, and compounds used to prepare and package meat and poultry products, the plants and equipment used, and processing techniques such as plant sanitation and thermal processing. It also regulates labeling of meat products. A research unit of FSIS develops and improves analytical procedures for detecting microbial and chemical adulterants and infectious and toxic agents in meat and poultry. FSIS has expanded its scope in recent years to encompass meat and poultry products from farm to table. Their work now includes examining farms, processing, transportation, distribution, storage, and retail establishments. The meat and poultry hotline, which offers information about how to handle, prepare, and store meat and poultry, is one of the ways FSIS is reaching out to consumers.

A comprehensive website offers consumer information, HACCP implementation procedures, and agency data.

United States Centers for Disease Control and Prevention (CDC)
1600 Clifton Road NE
Atlanta, GA 30333
Phone: (404) 639-3311
Website: http://www.cdc.gov

The mission of the Centers for Disease Control and Prevention is to promote health and quality of life by preventing and controlling disease, injury, and disability. As part of this mission, the CDC studies, monitors, researches diseases, and educates health practitioners and the public about foodborne illness. The CDC is often called in by state health departments to help trace and isolate the cause of foodborne illness outbreaks. Increasingly, the CDC is sending teams all over the world to assist with disease prevention because food and people travel, bringing disease across international boundaries.

In addition to background information about the CDC, a traveler's health link on the website gives information about health hazards and prevention in various parts of the world, Health Topics A-Z has information about many illnesses including foodborne ones, and a data and statistics link gives information about particular disease statistics.

United States Environmental Protection Agency (EPA)
401 M Street SW
Washington, DC 20460
Phone: (888) 372-8255
Website: http://www.epa.gov

The Environmental Protection Agency contributes to food safety by regulating the use of chemicals that affect people and the environment, including pesticide use. Recently USEPA has changed the way pesticide exposure is calculated. Under the new system, exposure to chemicals from all sources is calculated to determine acceptable levels. The Office of Child Protection of the EPA monitors pesticide exposure to children, and acceptable pesticide levels were recently recalculated to account for children's smaller bodies, immature development, and high food consumption relative to body weight. The Endocrine Disrupters Research Initiative is sponsored by USEPA to study whether certain chemicals that are present in the environment and that have the ability to interact with the endocrine system cause health problems. Some of these chemicals get into food from pesticides and drug residues found in animal products.

The website contains information about the activities of USEPA and links to other related sites.

International Agencies

Codex Alimentarius Commission
Executive Officer for Codex
U.S. Codex Contact Point
Food Safety and Inspection Service
U.S. Department of Agriculture
Room 4861 South Building
1400 Independence Avenue SW
Washington, DC 20250-3700
Phone: (202) 205-7760
Fax: (202) 720-3157

The Codex Alimentarius Commission was established in 1963 jointly by the World Health Organization and the Food and Agriculture Organization to set international food standards aimed at enabling trade and protecting consumers. The commission has developed more than two hundred standards for individual foods or groups of foods. It has also produced general standards for labeling of prepackaged foods, food hygiene, food additives, contaminants and toxins in food, irradiated food, maximum residue limits for pesticides and veterinary drugs, maximum limits for food additives and contaminants, and guidelines for nutrition labeling. Members of the Codex Alimentarius Commission include government officials, members of trade organizations, businesspeople, and representatives of consumer groups.

Food and Agricultural Organization of the United Nations (FAO)
Economic and Social Department
Food and Nutrition Division
Viale delle Terme di Caracalla
00100 Rome, Italy
Website: www.fao.org

The Food and Nutrition Division assesses and monitors the nutritional status of people all over the world and provides assistance and advice to improve nutrition for all. FAO devotes many of its resources to helping the poor and vulnerable in developing countries. Food safety and standards, food quality, and food science are active programs of FAO, and it sponsors research, disseminates information, and sponsors conferences in these areas. FAO cosponsors with the World Health Organization the Codex Alimentarius Commission (see above), the international standards-setting body that regulates food sold internationally.

Information about FAO's activities including conferences, as well as nutrition data, food composition, nutritional requirements, and food safety documents, are available on the website.

World Health Organization (WHO)
Liaison Office in Washington
1775 K Street NW, Suite 430
Washington, DC 20006
Phone: (202) 331-9081
Fax: (202) 331-9097
Website: http://www.who.int

The World Health Organization (WHO) was founded in 1948. A specialized agency of the UN, WHO promotes technical cooperation for health among nations, and carries out programs to control and eradicate disease. Hundreds of millions of people suffer from communicable diseases caused by contaminated food and water, and foodborne diseases are one of the major causes of malnutrition. WHO's safety program works to improve monitoring and control of foodborne hazards to reduce the incidence of disease. WHO also cosponsors with FAO the Codex Alimentarius Commission, the international food standards-setting body.

The website provides program and health information.

State Organizations

Each state has a different organizational structure that handles food safety concerns. Below is a list organized by state of the agencies within the state that address food safety issues. Most of these state agencies have websites. The websites can be found by using the following formula: http://www.state.(two-letter

abbreviation of state).us. For example: Alaska's website is http://www.state.ak.us.

Alaska

Environmental Sanitation/Food Safety Program
State Department of Environmental Conservation
610 University Avenue
Fairbanks, AK 99709-3643
Phone: (907) 451-2360
Fax: (907) 451-2188

Section of Epidemiology
Division of Public Health
State Department of Health and Social Services
3601 "C," Suite 540
Anchorage, AK 99519-6333
Phone: (907) 269-8000
Fax: (907) 561-6588

Arizona

Food Safety and Environmental Services
Arizona Department of Health Services
3815 North Black Canyon Highway
Phoenix, AZ 85015-5351
Phone: (602) 230-5917

Infectious Disease/Epidemiology Section
Arizona Department of Health Services
3815 North Black Canyon Highway
Phoenix, AZ 85015-5351
Phone: (602) 230-5800

Arkansas

Division of Health Maintenance
Bureau of Public Health Programs
State Department of Health
State Health Building
4815 Markham

Little Rock, AR 72205-3867
Phone: (501) 661-2227

Food Protection Services
Division of Environmental Health Protection
Bureau of Environmental Health Services
State Department of Health
State Health Building
4815 Markham
Little Rock, AR 72205-3867
Phone: (501) 661-2171
Fax: (501) 661-2572

California

Environmental Health/Investigations Branch (Epidemiology)
5900 Hollis Street, Suite E
Emeryville, CA 94608
Phone: (510) 450-3818

State Department of Food and Agriculture
1220 N Street, P.O. Box 942871
Sacramento, CA 94271
Phone: (916) 654-0433
Fax: (916) 654-0403

Includes the Division of Inspection Services, which monitors feeds, fertilizers, and livestock drugs.

State Department of Health Services
Division of Food, Drug, and Radiation Safety
601 N. Seventh Avenue
P.O. Box 942732
Sacramento, CA 94232-7320
Phone: (916) 324-3266

State Environmental Protection Agency
Department of Pesticide Regulation
1020 N Street, Room 100
Sacramento, CA 95814
Phone: (916) 445-4000
Fax: (916) 324-1452

Colorado

Disease Surveillance Section
Division of Disease Control and Environmental
   Epidemiology
Colorado Department of Public Health and Environment
4300 Cherry Creek Drive South
Denver, CO 80222-1530
Phone: (303) 692-2662

Food Protection Program
Division of Consumer Protection
4300 Cherry Creek Drive South
Denver, CO 80222-1530
Phone: (303) 692-2662

Connecticut

Food Division
State Department of Consumer Protection
State Office Building
165 Capitol Avenue
Hartford, CT 06106
Phone: (860) 566-3388

Food Protection Program
Environmental Health Division
State Department of Community Health
410 Capitol Avenue
P.O. Box 340308
Hartford, CT 06134-0308
Phone: (860) 509-7297

Infectious Disease Division
Bureau of Community Health
State Department of Community Health
410 Capitol Avenue
P.O. Box 340308
Hartford, CT 06134-0308
Phone: (860) 509-7995

Delaware

Epidemiology Branch
Delaware Public Health
Administration Building
Delaware State Hospital
1901 North Dupont Highway
New Castle, DE 19720
Phone: (302) 739-3033

Food Products Inspection and Pesticides
Department of Agriculture
2320 South Dupont Highway
Dover, DE 19901
Phone: (302) 739-4811

Office of Food Protection
Delaware Public Health
Administration Building
Delaware State Hospital
1901 North Dupont Highway
New Castle, DE 19720
Phone: (302) 739-3841

District of Columbia

Food Protection Branch
Department of Consumer and Regulatory Affairs
614 H Street NW
Washington, DC 20001
Phone: (202) 727-7250
Fax: (202) 727-8030

Preventive Health Services Administration
Department of Human Services
800 9th Street SW
Washington, DC 20024
Phone: (202) 645-5544
Fax: (202) 645-0536

Florida

Division of Food Safety
Agriculture and Consumer Services
Laboratory Complex
3125 Conner Boulevard
Tallahassee, FL 32399-1650
Phone: (850) 488-0295
Fax: (850) 488-7946

Epidemiology
State Department of Health
1323 Winewood Boulevard
Tallahassee, FL 32301
Mailing Address:
1317 Winewood Boulevard
Tallahassee, FL 32399-0700
Phone: (850) 922-2203
Fax: (850) 922-9299

Georgia

Consumer Protection Field Forces Division
State Department of Agriculture
19 Martin Luther King Drive SW
Atlanta, GA 30334-2001
Phone: (404) 656-3621
Fax: (404) 656-9380

Epidemiology/Prevention Branch
Division of Public Health
2 Peachtree Street NE
Atlanta, GA 30303
Phone: (404) 657-2588
Fax: (404) 657-2586

Hawaii

Communicable Disease Division
Department of Health
591 Ala Moana Boulevard
Honolulu, HI 96813

Phone: (808) 586-4580
Fax: (808) 586-4729

Quality Assurance Division
State Department of Agriculture
1428 S. King Street
Honolulu, HI 96814
Mailing Address:
P.O. Box 22159
Honolulu, HI 96823-0159
Phone: (808) 973-9566
Fax: (808) 973-0880

Idaho

Food Protection Program
Epidemiological Programs
Bureau of Environmental Health and Safety
Idaho Department of Health and Welfare
450 W. State Street
P.O. Box 83720
Boise, ID 83720-0036
Food Protection: (208) 334-5938
Epidemiology: (208) 334-5939

Illinois

Division of Infectious Disease
825 N. Rutledge
Springfield, IL 62794
Phone: (217) 782-2016

Food Section
Division of Food, Drugs, and Dairies
State Department of Public Health
525 W. Jefferson
Springfield, IL 62761
Phone: (217) 785-2439
Fax: (217) 524-0802

Indiana

Chronic/Communicable Disease/Immunization
Indiana State Department of Health
2 North Meridian Street
Indianapolis, IN 46204
Phone: (317) 233-7467
Fax: (317) 383-6776

Food Protection
Indiana State Department of Health
2 North Meridian Street
Indianapolis, IN 46204
Phone: (317) 233-7164

Iowa

Epidemiology
Department of Public Health
Lucas State Office Building
Des Moines, IA 50319
Phone: (515) 281-4941

Food and Consumer Safety Bureau
State Department of Inspections and Appeals
Lucas State Office Building, Second Floor
Des Moines, IA 50319
Phone: (515) 281-6539
Fax: (515) 281-3291

Kansas

Office of Epidemiology
Department of Health and Environment
Landon State Office Building
900 SW Jackson Street
Topeka, KS 66612
Phone: (913) 296-6536
Fax: (913) 291-3775

Food Protection Program
Bureau of Environmental Health Services
109 SW 9th Street, Suite 604
Topeka, KS 66612
Phone: (913) 296-5599
Fax: (913) 296-6522

Kentucky

Division of Epidemiology
Department of Health Services
275 E. Main Street
Frankfort, KY 40621
Phone: (502) 564-7130
Fax: (502) 564-7573

Food Safety and Cosmetics Branch
Department of Health Services
275 E. Main Street
Frankfort, KY 40621
Phone: (502) 564-7181
Fax: (502) 564-7573

Louisiana

Epidemiology Section
Division of Laboratories
Office of Public Health
325 Loyola Avenue
P.O. Box 60630
New Orleans, LA 70160
Phone: (504) 568-5005
Fax: (504) 568-3206

Food and Drug Unit
Office of Public Health
325 Loyola Avenue
P.O. Box 60630
New Orleans, LA 70160
Phone: (504) 568-5401
Fax: (504) 568-8102

Maine

Eating and Lodging Program
Bureau of Health
221 State Street
Augusta, ME
Mailing Address:
State House Station 11
Augusta, ME 04333
Phone: (207) 287-5693
Fax: (207) 287-4172

Epidemiology
Bureau of Health
221 State Street
Augusta, ME
Mailing Address:
State House Station 11
Augusta, ME 04333
Phone: (207) 287-3591

Food Program/Division of Quality Assurance
Department of Agriculture
Food and Rural Resources
Deering Building
Augusta, ME
Mailing Address:
State House Station 28
Augusta, ME 04333
Phone: (207) 287-3481

Maryland

Division of Food Control
State Department of Health and Mental Hygiene
201 W. Preston Street (7th Floor Mailroom)
Baltimore, MD 21201
Phone: (410) 225-6700
Fax: (410) 669-4215

Epidemiology
State Department of Health and Mental Hygiene

201 W. Preston Street (7th Floor Mailroom)
Baltimore, MD 21201
Phone: (410) 225-6700
Fax: (410) 669-4215

Massachusetts

Division of Epidemiology
State Department of Public Health
305 South Street
Jamaica Plain, MA 02130
Phone: (617) 983-6800

Division of Food and Drugs
State Department of Public Health
305 South Street
Jamaica Plain, MA 02130
Phone: (617) 983-6759
Fax: (617) 524-8062

Michigan

Bureau of Epidemiology
State Department of Community Health
3500 N. Martin Luther King Boulevard
Lansing, MI 48906
Phone: (517) 335-9218

Food Division
State Department of Agriculture
611 W. Ottawa
P.O. Box 30017
Lansing, MI 48909
Phone: (517) 373-1060
Fax: (517) 373-3333

Minnesota

Dairy and Food Inspection Division
State Department of Agriculture
90 W. Plato Boulevard
St. Paul, MN 55107

Phone: (612) 296-2629
Fax: (612) 297-5637

Epidemiology
State Health Department
State Department of Health Building
121 E. 7th Place, Suite 450
P.O. Box 64975
St. Paul, MN 55164
Phone: (612) 623-5414

Mississippi

Food Vector Control and General Sanitation Branch
P.O. Box 1700
2423 N. State Street
Jackson, MS 39215
Phone: (601) 960-7725
Fax: (601) 960-7909

Office of Community Health Services
P.O. Box 1700
2423 N. State Street
Jackson, MS 39215
Phone: (601) 960-7725
Fax: (601) 960-7909

Missouri

Food Protection and Processing
Bureau of Community Environmental Health
930 Wildwood Drive
Jefferson City, MO 65102
Phone: (573) 751-6095

Office of Epidemiology Services
Division of Environmental Health and Communicable Disease
    Prevention
State Department of Health
920 Wildwood Drive
P.O. Box 570

Jefferson City, MO 65102
Phone: (573) 751-6128

Montana

Food and Consumer Safety
Health Policy and Services Division
Montana Department of Public Health and Human Services
1400 Broadway
Helena, MT 59620
Phone: (406) 444-4540

Nebraska

Bureau of Dairies and Food
State Department of Agriculture
301 Centennial Mall S
P.O. Box 95064
Lincoln, NE 68509
Phone: (402) 471-2536
Fax: (402) 471-3252

Epidemiology
State Department of Health and Human Services Regulation
    and Licensure
301 Centennial Mall S
P.O. Box 95007
Lincoln, NE 68509

Nevada

Bureau of Health Protection Services
State Department of Human Resources
505 E. King Street, Room 600
Carson City, NV 89701
Phone: (702) 687-4750
Fax: (702) 687-5197

The Bureau of Health Protection Services handles both epidemiology and food safety concerns.

New Hampshire

Bureau of Disease Control (Epidemiology)
State Department of Health and Human Services
Health and Welfare Building
6 Hazen Drive
Concord, NH 03301
Phone: (603) 271-4477

Bureau of Food Protection
State Department of Health and Human Services
Health and Welfare Building
6 Hazen Drive
Concord, NH 03301
Phone: (603) 271-4583

New Jersey

**Division of Epidemiology and
Communicable Disease Control**
State Department of Health
Health Agriculture Building
John Fitch Plaza
Trenton, NJ 08625
Mailing Address:
CN 369
Trenton, NJ 08625
Phone: (609) 588-7463

Food and Milk Program
State Department of Health
Health Agriculture Building
John Fitch Plaza
Trenton, NJ 08625
Mailing Address:
CN 369
Trenton, NJ 08625
Phone: (609) 588-3123

New Mexico

Food Program
State Department of Environment
4131 Montgomery Boulevard
Albuquerque, NM 87109
Phone: (505) 841-9450
Fax: (505) 884-9254

Public Health Division (Epidemiology)
State Department of Health
1190 St. Francis Drive
Santa Fe, NM 87505
Phone: (505) 827-0006

New York

Bureau of Communicable Disease Control
State Department of Health
Tower Building
Empire State Plaza
Albany, NY 12237
Phone: (518) 473-4436

Food Protection Section
State Department of Health
2 University Place
Albany, NY 12203
Phone: (518) 458-6706

North Carolina

Epidemiology Section
State Department of Environment, Health, and Natural
  Resources
512 N. Salisbury Street
P.O. Box 27687
Raleigh, NC 27611
Phone: (919) 733-3419
Fax: (919) 733-0490

Food and Drug Protection Division
4000 Reedy Creek Road
Raleigh, NC 27607
Phone: (919) 733-7366
Fax: (919) 733-6801

North Dakota

Division of Food and Lodging
State Department of Health
600 E. Boulevard Avenue
Bismarck, ND 58505
Phone: (701) 328-1291
Fax: (701) 328-1412

Epidemiology
Division of Disease Control
State Department of Health
600 E. Boulevard Avenue
Bismarck, ND 58505
Phone: (701) 328-2378
Fax: (701) 328-1412

Ohio

Bureau of Epidemiology
State Department of Health
246 N. High Street
P.O. Box 118
Columbus, OH 43266
Phone: (614) 466-4643

Division of Foods, Dairies, and Drugs
State Department of Agriculture
Broomfield Administration Building
8995 E. Main Street
Reynoldsburg, OH 43068
Phone: (614) 728-6250
Fax: (614) 728-4235

Food Protection Unit
Division of Environmental Health

246 N. High Street
P.O. Box 118
Columbus, OH 43266
Phone: (614) 466-5190

Oklahoma

Environmental Health Services
State Department of Health
1000 NE 10th Street
Oklahoma City, OK 73117
Phone: (405) 271-5217
Fax: (405) 271-3458

Epidemiology
State Department of Health
1000 NE 10th Street
Oklahoma City, OK 73117
Phone: (405) 271-3266
Fax: (405) 271-1166

Oregon

Center for Disease Prevention and Epidemiology
Health Division
800 NE Oregon Street, Suite 925
P.O. Box 14450
Portland, OR 97214-0450
Phone: (503) 731-4023

Food Safety Division
Oregon Department of Agriculture
Agriculture Building
635 Capitol Street NE
Salem, OR 97310-0110
Phone: (503) 986-4720

Pennsylvania

Bureau of Epidemiology
State Department of Health
Health and Welfare Building

7th & Forster Streets
P.O. Box 90
Harrisburg, PA 17108
Phone: (717) 787-3350

Bureau of Food Safety and Laboratory Services
State Department of Agriculture
2301 N. Cameron Street
Harrisburg, PA 17110
Phone: (717) 787-4315
Fax: (717) 772-2780

Rhode Island

Disease Control (Epidemiology)
State Department of Health
3 Capitol Hill
Providence, RI 02908
Phone: (401) 277-1171

Office of Food Protection
State Department of Health
3 Capitol Hill
Providence, RI 02908
Phone: (401) 277-2750
Fax: (401) 277-6953

South Carolina

Bureau of Preventative Health Services (Epidemiology)
State Department of Health and Environmental Control
J. Marion Sims Building
2600 Bull Street
Columbia, SC 29201
Phone: (803) 737-4040
Fax: (803) 737-4036

Division of Food Protection
Bureau of Environmental Health
State Department of Health and Environmental Control
J. Marion Sims Building

2600 Bull Street
Columbia, SC 29201
Phone: (803) 935-7958
Fax: (803) 935-7825

South Dakota

Disease Prevention/Epidemiology
State Department of Health
Anderson Building
445 E. Capitol Avenue
Pierre, SD 57501
Phone: (605) 773-3361
Fax: (605) 773-5683

Division of Health Systems Development/Regulation
State Department of Health
Anderson Building
445 E. Capitol Avenue
Pierre, SD 57501
Phone: (605) 773-3364
Fax: (605) 773-5904

Tennessee

Division of Quality and Standards
State Department of Agriculture
Ellington Agricultural Center
P.O. Box 40627
Nashville, TN 37204
Phone: (615) 360-0155
Fax: (615) 360-0335

Epidemiology
State Department of Health
426 5th Avenue N
Nashville, TN 37247
Phone: (615) 741-7247

Texas

Bureau of Food and Drug Safety
State Department of Health
100 W. 49th Street
Austin, TX 78746
Phone: (512) 719-0222
Fax: (512) 719-0202

Disease Control and Prevention/Epidemiology
State Department of Health
100 W. 49th Street
Austin, TX 78746
Phone: (512) 458-7729
Fax: (512) 458-7229

Utah

Bureau of Epidemiology
State Department of Health
46 N. Medical Drive
Salt Lake City, UT 84113
Phone: (801) 538-6191
Fax: (801) 538-6036

Food Program Specialist
Bureau of Environmental Services
288 N. 1460 West
Salt Lake City, UT 84114
Phone: (801) 538-6755
Fax: (801) 538-6036

Vermont

Environmental Health Division
State Department of Health
108 Cherry Street
P.O. Box 70
Burlington, VT 05402
Phone: (802) 863-7220

Epidemiology
State Department of Health
108 Cherry Street
P.O. Box 70
Burlington, VT 05402
Phone: (802) 863-7240

Virginia

Division of Food/Environmental Services
State Department of Health
1500 E. Main Street, Room 214
P.O. Box 2448
Richmond, VA 23218
Phone: (804) 786-1750
Fax: (804) 225-4003

Office of Epidemiology
State Department of Health
1500 E. Main Street, Room 214
P.O. Box 2448
Richmond, VA 23218
Phone: (804) 786-6029
Fax: (804) 786-1076

Washington

Communicable Disease Control Section
State Department of Health
1610 NE 150th Street
Seattle, WA 98155-9701
Phone: (206) 361-2831

Food Safety and Animal Health Division
Washington State Department of Agriculture
1111 Washington Street
P.O. Box 42560
Olympia, WA 98504-2560
Phone: (360) 902-1800

West Virginia

Division of Surveillance and Disease Control
Bureau of Public Health
1422 Washington Street East
Charleston, WV 25301
Phone: (304) 558-5358
Fax: (304) 558-6335

Environmental Health Services
Bureau of Public Health
815 Quarrier Street
Charleston, WV 25301
Phone: (304) 558-2981
Fax: (304) 558-1291

Wisconsin

Division of Food Safety
Department of Agriculture, Trade, and Consumer Protection
2811 Agriculture Drive
P.O. Box 8911
Madison, WI 53708
Phone: (608) 224-4701
Fax: (608) 224-4710

Epidemiology
Bureau of Public Health
1414 E. Washington Avenue
P.O. Box 309
Madison, WI 53701
Phone: (608) 297-9003

Wyoming

Division of Consumer Health Services
State Department of Agriculture
2219 Carey Avenue
Cheyenne, WY 82002
Phone: (307) 777-6591
Fax: (307) 777-6593

This department is responsible for both epidemiology and food safety.

6

Print Resources

There are many helpful books and journals for studying food safety issues. The books below were chosen based on currency, ideas, and accessibility to general readers. Older books were included if the ideas they presented were unique and their research was still pertinent. At the end of this chapter is a listing of magazines and journals that are specifically about food safety or consistently offer food safety articles. Many other magazines and journals present food safety articles occasionally. The databases listed in the nonprint resources section will allow more focused searching in articles ranging from the general to the technical. The books are divided into topics to make it easier to find appropriate materials.

Books

Reference Works. This section includes dictionaries, encyclopedias, indexes, and manuals about food safety.

Animal Products. Animal products are the foods most likely to carry foodborne disease and have the highest levels of pesticide and drug residues. The books in this section discuss the hazards of animal products and ways to keep animal products safe.

Consumer Resources. These books are directed specifically at consumers with information about safe food handling, storing, cooking, and avoiding foodborne illness.

Courses. There are several professional food safety certification courses. These works prepare the reader for the certification exams.

Food Additives. The safety of chemicals added intentionally to food is discussed in these books.

Food Safety in Commercial Applications. These books offer technical details of implementing HACCP plans.

Food Safety Law and Policy. Some of the works in this section offer theory about how food policy should be implemented; other works are more practical.

Foodborne Diseases. These works are specifically about food-borne illness.

General. General works on food safety not specifically geared toward consumers are in this section.

Genetically Modified Foods. Biotechnology has changed the way many foods are produced. These books discuss the safety of genetically modified products.

History. These works describe how food safety legislation came about.

Irradiation and Other Methods of Preservation. Besides irradiation, there are many traditional and new preservation methods discussed in the books in this section.

Microbiology of Foods. The role microorganisms play in food spoilage, food production, food preservation, and foodborne disease is covered by the term "food microbiology."

Pesticides. Safety of pesticides and how to avoid foods with the most pesticides are included in this section.

Toxins and Contaminants. These works cover a range of toxins and contaminants, from naturally occurring to environmental hazards.

Reference Works

Bartone, Mary. *Food and Its Dangerous Ingredients for Health and Safety in America.* Washington, DC: ABBE Publishers, 1995. 179p. ISBN 0788307568 (case), $47.50; ISBN 0788307576 (paper), $44.50.

This index is designed to help locate references on the health consequences of food ingredients. Both author and subject indexes provide access to scholarly articles.

Frank, Hanns. *Dictionary of Food Microbiology.* Lancaster, PA: Technomic Publishing, 1992. 298p. ISBN 0566760100, $89.95.

This useful dictionary of mostly technical terms features longish entries, British spellings, and references at the end of the book.

Furia, Thomas. *CRC Handbook of Food Additives,* Volume II. Boca Raton, FL: CRC Press, 1980. 998p. ISBN 0849305438, $220.95.

This scientific treatment covers chemical structure of food additives, including antioxidants as stabilizers for fats, oils, and lipid-containing foods; enzymes; nonnutritive sweeteners: saccharin, cyclamates, and other sweeteners; and natural and artificial colors and flavors. A section covers the legal considerations of food additives.

Hui, Y. H., ed. *Encyclopedia of Food Science and Technology.* 4 volumes. New York: John Wiley and Sons, 1992. ISBN 0471505412. Out of print.

Contains 380 signed articles on topics such as toxicology, sanitation, foodborne diseases, HACCP. Each entry is six to seven pages long and contains references, diagrams, and charts.

Lewis, Richard. *Food Additives Handbook.* New York: Chapman and Hall, 1989. 592p. ISBN 0442205082, $105.

An introduction discusses the regulatory status of food additives and their use by the food industry. The bulk of the book is arranged in encyclopedic format and includes the molecular formula, properties, synonyms, purpose, where used, regulations applicable to the additive, cancer reviews, status of National Toxicology Program testing, EPA Extremely Hazardous Substances list, Community Right to Know list, and the EPA Genetic Toxicology program, standards, and safety profiles. Well indexed with purpose served in food index, food type, Chemical Abstract Registry Number, and synonyms indexes.

Robinson, Richard, Carl Batt, and Pradip Patel, eds. *Encyclopedia of Food Microbiology.* 3 volumes. San Diego, CA: Academic Press, 2000. ISBN 0122270703 (set), $925.

Three hundred fifty-eight articles cover important groups of bacteria, fungi, parasites, and viruses; methods for detection in foods; factors that govern the behavior of these organisms; and likely outcomes of microbial growth and metabolism in terms of disease and spoilage. This work also includes beneficial microorganisms for industrial fermentation, including traditional food fermentation from the Middle and Far East and production of fermented foods like bread, cheese, and yogurt. This is an exceptionally well-organized encyclopedia. The table of contents provides references to all articles where the topic occurs, "see also" references are included both in the text of articles and as entries, and there are lots of illustrations, charts, tables, and color plates.

Salunkhe, D. K., H. R. Bolin, and N. R. Reddy. *Storage Processing and Nutritional Quality of Fruits and Vegetables.* Boca Raton, FL: CRC Press, 1991. ISBN 0849356237 (case); ISBN 0849356245 (paper). Out of print.

This scientifically based work covers fresh product handling, preparation of preserved products, identification of disease organisms, insect identification, physiological disorders, and nutritional values. Chemical composition and nutritional quality, chemical changes during ripening and storage, development of postharvest diseases, postharvest entomology, storage methods, transportation, distribution, and marketing are included for each fruit and vegetable.

Talbot, Ross B. *Historical Dictionary of the International Food Agencies: FAO, WFP, WFC, IFAD.* Metuchen, NJ: Scarecrow Press, 1994. 169p. ISBN 0810828472, $35.

This dictionary has detailed entries and chronologies of the major international food agencies, as well as organizational charts and tables. The dictionary is arranged by agency. Although not limited to food safety issues, this dictionary can help the reader identify the specific roles each agency plays in international food safety.

United States Government Department of Health and Human Services. *United States Food Code.* Washington, DC: National Technical Information Service, U.S. Department of Commerce, 1999. 432p. ISBN 0934213682, $40.

The complete Food Code has been updated jointly by the Food and Drug Administration, Food Safety and Inspection Service of the USDA, and the Centers for Disease Control and Prevention in collaboration with the Conference for Food Protection, state and local officials, consumers, industry representatives, and academics. The current version of the code has been rewritten to explain precautions that should be taken to prevent specific foodborne illnesses. An interesting feature of the code is that explanations are given for regulations.

United States Government, Food and Drug Administration. *A Food Labeling Guide.* Washington, DC: U.S. Department of Health and Human Services, Public Health Service, 1994. 65p. ISBN 0160452120, $6.

In a question-and-answer format, the food labeling rules are explained. The guide explains how certain claims must be displayed on the label, how to calculate serving sizes, the size of the type that must be used to describe products, and when to use the word "imitation."

Wilkinson, V. M., and G. W. Gould. *Food Irradiation: A Reference Guide.* Cambridge, U.K.: Woodhead Publishing, 1996. 177p. ISBN 1855733595, $126.

In dictionary format with references, each entry covers a food or property, terms related to irradiation, statistics, and diagrams. A useful and comprehensive work on irradiation.

Animal Products

Cohen, Robert. *Milk: The Deadly Poison.* Englewood Cliffs, NJ: Argus Publishing, 1998. 317pp. ISBN 0965919609 (case), $24.95; ISBN 0965919617 (paper), $14.95.

In this self-published work, the author expresses his belief that the current high levels of milk consumption are responsible for the prevalence of cancer in this country because the pasteurization process does not kill the natural and artificial hormones present in milk. The author describes the adoption of recombinant bovine growth hormone (rBGH) and other hazards in milk. Very poorly organized.

Committee on Drug Use in Food Animals; Panel on Animal Health, Food Safety, and Public Health; Board on Agriculture, National Research Council; Food and Nutrition Council, Institute of Medicine. *Use of Drugs in Food Animals: Benefits and Risks.* Washington, DC: National Academy Press, 1999. 253p. $34.95.

After reviewing the use of drugs in food animals since 1970, this work covers current production practices, benefits and hazards to human health from animal drug use, development of new drugs including the approval process, description of current drug residue monitoring programs, antibiotic resistance, economic implications of eliminating antibiotics in subtherapeutic doses, alternative strategies to reduce the need for drug use, and promising areas of research. Recommendations are offered for improving drug-resistance monitoring, drug-residue monitoring, and developing alternative strategies to drug use.

Gil, J. Infante, and J. Costa Durao. *A Colour Atlas of Meat Inspection.* London: Wolfe Publishing, 1990. 453p. ISBN 0723407088, $77.

This atlas, intended for those working as meat inspectors or studying animal pathology, features pictures that have been collected over more than twenty years and cover most pathological conditions likely to occur in day-to-day meat inspection, both before and after slaughter. A few of the pictures involve cases of natural death. Each picture caption describes the condition, gives other conditions likely to be present, and makes recommendations based on the International Code of Practice for Ante-Mortem and Post-Mortem Judgment of Slaughter Animals and Meat.

Hubbert, William, et al. *Food Safety and Quality Assurance: Foods of Animal Origin,* 2nd ed. Ames: Iowa State University, 1996. 305p. ISBN 081380714X, $44.95.

This textbook is designed to prepare students to identify human health hazards in food of animal origin; the role of veterinarians in preventing health hazards from entering the food chain; government and private-sector organizations and their role in improving food safety; principles of safe food production, processing, and handling; and data collection and analysis techniques for investigation of foodborne disease outbreaks. Includes information about laws and processes around the world.

Hulse, Virgil. *Mad Cows and Milk Gate.* Phoenix, OR: Marble Mountain Publishing, 1996. 286p. ISBN 0965437701, $20.

The author, a medical doctor and former milk inspector, believes that milk and dairy products cause cancer. He notes that bovine leukemia virus is not controlled in the United States. (Milk cannot be sold in Europe if it contains the virus.) Further, he states that excess fat in the diet does not cause cancer as many scientists believe, but rather fat is generally consumed in high quantities with dairy products and is a confounding factor. He believes retroviruses in meat and dairy products cause cancer. Includes a thorough timeline of bovine spongiform encephalopathy (BSE).

Lyman, Howard, and Glen Merzer. *Mad Cowboy: Plain Truth from the Cattle Rancher Who Won't Eat Meat.* New York: Scribner, 1998. 223p. ISBN 0684845164, $23.

Lyman was a fourth-generation Montana dairy farmer and cattle rancher who ran a feedlot for twenty years. A serious illness prompted him to rethink the chemical farming methods he was using. He was a guest on the Oprah Winfrey Show and was sued with Winfrey for food disparagement in 1996. In this highly readable account, Lyman discusses mad cow disease; recombinant bovine growth hormone (rBGH), the synthetic hormone used to boost milk production; and the effect of chemical agriculture on the environment. He tells his own story of how he went from cattle rancher to president of the International Vegetarian Union.

Robbins, John. *Diet for a New America.* Walpole, NH: Stillpoint Publishing, 1987. 423p. ISBN 0913299545 (paper), $13.95.

Robbins, a vegetarian activist, describes scientific studies showing the detrimental effects on human health caused by eating animal products, such as higher rates of cancer, heart disease, osteoporosis, and diabetes. The bioaccumulation of pesticides in meat and dairy products, environmental consequences of meat production, and humanitarian aspects of factory farming are also discussed.

Schell, Orville. *Modern Meat.* New York: Random House, 1984. 337p. ISBN 039451890X, $17.95.

Modern livestock production includes many practices that are vastly different from the techniques used at the beginning of the twentieth century. Schell, a farmer, investigates antibiotic feed additives, animal feed technologies, and hormonal compounds. Antibiotic use became widespread in the mid-1960s on a subtherapeutic level to treat diseases that do not show evident symptoms, but nevertheless tax the animal, and to promote growth in almost all commercially raised meat animals. Foodstuffs have similarly changed to increase efficiency. Plastic hay, cardboard, and garbage are all fed to livestock. Hormonal compounds are used to enhance cattle growth or to manipulate the reproductive system. Schell argues that many of these practices are not safe.

Consumer Resources

Acheson, David, and Robin Levinson. *Safe Eating: Protect Yourself against E. coli, Salmonella, and Other Deadly Food-Borne Pathogens.* New York: Dell, 1998. 333p. ISBN 044022659 (paper), $6.50.

Designed for the consumer, this guide explains how bacteria, viruses, and parasites can infiltrate food and drinking water; which foods are most vulnerable to biological hazards; what government and industry can and cannot do to protect individuals from foodborne infections; why certain people are at high risk of contracting the most common foodborne illnesses; how to determine whether you're at risk for foodborne illness; why *Escherichia coli* O157:H7 is among the most deadly; how infectious agents harm the human body; which treatments help; when to seek medical attention; how to help a doctor diagnose a foodborne disease; and how to reduce the risk of eating contaminated foods.

Elder, Joseph. *Buy It Fresh, Keep It Fresh: The Complete A to Z Guide to Selecting and Storing Food.* New York: Fawcett, 1990. 149p. ISBN 0449146405. Out of print.

In dictionary format, each entry describes a particular food and how to tell if it is fresh, how to store it, and how long it can be stored.

Fox, Nicols. *It Was Probably Something You Ate: A Practical Guide to Avoiding and Surviving a Foodborne Illness.* New York: Penguin, 1999. 229p. ISBN 0140277994, $13.95.

Fox describes the major foodborne illnesses with descriptions of particular outbreaks and poisonings along with facts about each disease. How to eat out and travel; how to buy, store, and prepare foods; how to survive a foodborne illness as an adult; the WHO rehydration formula; children and foodborne illness; and what action should be taken by government are discussed. Includes resources and a bibliography.

Garland, Anne Witte. *For Our Kids' Sake: How to Protect Your Child against Pesticides in Food.* San Francisco: Sierra Club Books, 1989. 87p. ISBN 0871566133. Out of print.

Divided into three sections, the problem, solutions, and tools, this is an effective summary of the dangers of pesticide use, what the government and individuals can do to reduce pesticide exposure, and a list of resources and action steps to take. A summary of the pesticides commonly applied to the produce children eat is included.

Goodman, Robert. *A Quick Guide to Food Safety.* San Diego, CA: Silvercat Publications, 1992. 86p. ISBN 0962494534 (paper), $6.95.

The focus of this work is food additives. More than three thousand chemicals are used in the average diet, including pesticides, hormones, antibiotics, packaging chemicals, industrial contaminants, and natural contaminants. More than half of the typical American diet is processed or packaged and contains significant food additives. The author concludes that additives dilute quality, and items with additives usually cost more than the item would cost prepared at home from scratch. A dictionary of common additives and a strategy for minimizing food additive consumption is included.

Jacobson, Michael, Lisa Lefferts, and Anne Witte Garland, Center for Science in the Public Interest. *Safe Food: Eating Wisely in a Risky World.* Venice, CA: Living Planet Press, 1991. 234p. ISBN 1879326019 (paper), $9.95; ISBN 0425136213 (paper), $4.99.

Overall eating guidelines as well as specific chapters that describe safely choosing and preparing fruits and vegetables, seafood, meats, dairy products, and nuts and grains. This commonsense guide includes procedures for having a safe kitchen and a chapter of ways to be politically active to increase food safety.

Lehmann, Robert. *Cooking for Life: A Guide to Nutrition and Food Safety for the HIV Positive Community.* New York: Dell, 1997. 244p. ISBN 0440507537 (paper), $10.95.

Good nutrition is essential for surviving HIV on a long-term basis. This practical guide addresses preventing wasting, the ideal diet for health, cooking tips, and a very well-thought-out food safety section that includes shopping, cooking, using a bleach solution to keep the kitchen sanitized, and safely eating away from home. Although aimed at people who are HIV positive, the food safety section would be helpful for any high-risk individual.

Matthews, Dawn, ed. *Food Safety Sourcebook: Basic Consumer Information about the Safe Handling of Meat, Poultry, Seafood, Eggs, Fruit Juices, and Other Food Items and Facts about Pesticides, Drinking Water, Food Safety Overseas, and the Onset, Duration, and Symptoms of Foodborne Illnesses, Including Types of Pathogenic Bacteria, Parasitic Protozoa, Worms, Viruses, and Natural Toxins, along with the Role of the Consumer, the Food Handler, and the Government in Food Safety; a Glossary, and Resources for Additional Help and Information.* Detroit, MI: Omnigraphics, 1999. 339p. ISBN 0780803264, $48.

Designed for consumers handling food in their own kitchens and for workers in the food industry. A collection of articles reprinted from government and other sources.

Satin, Morton. *Food Alert: The Ultimate Sourcebook for Food Safety.* New York: Facts on File, 1999. 306p. ISBN 0816039356 (case), $27.95; ISBN 0816039364 (paper), $14.95.

Lots of charts, tables, checklists, and quizzes liven up this food safety book. Historical background, antibiotic resistance, and the twenty most common causes of foodborne illness in the kitchen comprise the first part of the book. Several chapters are divided by food type, including poultry, beef, dairy products, fish and shellfish, and fruits and vegetables. These chapters tell what kinds of hazards exist and how to avoid them. A helpful appendix lists disease causes and symptoms, safe food storage procedures, and information sources on foodborne diseases.

Scott, Elizabeth, and Paul Sockett. *How to Prevent Food Poisoning.* New York: John Wiley and Sons, 1998. 207p. ISBN 0471195766 (paper), $14.95.

Two scientists, Scott, a microbiologist specializing in consumer hygiene issues, and Sockett, a microbiologist and epidemiologist, have used their extensive training to explain how consumers can prevent food poisoning. Scott and Sockett state that the most common causes of food poisoning for consumers are allowing raw food to contaminate kitchen surfaces and failing to wash hands. In this well-organized guide, chapters explain how food poisoning happens; how to shop safely for food; how to prepare, cook, and store food in everyday home situations; and how to ensure food safety for higher-risk individuals. Also includes a glossary and descriptions of various foodborne illnesses.

Winter, Ruth. *Poisons in Your Food: The Dangers You Face and What You Can Do about Them.* New York: Crown Publishers, 1991. 321p. ISBN 0517576813, $10.95.

This book is a new edition of the work originally published in 1969. The author, a science writer, frequently compares what she wrote in 1969 to the state of affairs over twenty years later. Sadly, most of the dangers she wrote about in 1969 are still problems, and there are new challenges to food safety as well. Insecticides; additives; meat, poultry, and fish hazards; types of food poisoning; how to eat out; water; and new food technologies such as convenience foods and modified environment packaging are discussed. A well-researched and practical book.

Courses

Cichy, Ronald F. *Quality Sanitation Management.* East Lansing, MI: Educational Institute of the American Hotel and Motel Association, 1994. 448p. ISBN 086612084X, $61.95.

This work prepares the reader for the American Hotel and Motel Association food safety certificate exam. Based on the FDA's 1993 Food Code, it takes a systems approach to sanitation risk management. Topics include food spoilage and preservation; menu planning and purchasing; receiving, storing, and issuing; preparing, holding, and cooking; serving; and cleaning and maintenance of facilities. Includes review quizzes, a summary of pathogenic microorganisms, index, and glossary.

Educational Foundation of the National Restaurant Association. *ServSafe—Serving Safe Food Certification Coursebook.* Chicago, IL: Education Foundation of the National Restaurant Association, 1995. ISBN 1883904285, $72.

The ServSafe course is the leading food safety course in the United States. Starting with practical reasons to implement a food safety program, like avoiding lawsuits and keeping customers, this work outlines the elements of implementing a food safety plan from hazards, to HACCP, purchasing, receiving, storing, cleaning, sanitizing, and integrated pest management. Quizzes, bibliography, glossary, and index.

McSwane, David, Nancy Rue, and Richard Linton. *Essentials of Safe Food Management and Sanitation.* Upper Saddle River, NJ: Prentice Hall, 1997. 373p. ISBN 0135321360. Out of print.

This work prepares readers for the Certified Food Safety Manager exam, a two-hour test for food managers in restaurants and other food service operations. An easy-to-read book, topics include food safety and sanitation management, hazards to food safety, types of foodborne illnesses, factors that affect foodborne illness (e.g., temperature abuse and improper hand washing), proper procedures for receiving and storing food, HACCP, facilities cleaning and sanitizing, environmental sanitation and maintenance, food safety regulations, accident prevention and crisis management, and education and training. Quizzes, cartoons, and photographs throughout.

National Assessment Institute. *Handbook for Safe Food Service Management.* Upper Saddle River, NJ: Prentice Hall, 1998. 200p. ISBN 0132361183 (paper), $47.

This work prepares the reader for the national Certified Professional Food Manager (CPFM) exam. Intended to be a fifteen-hour course, the book covers managerial responsibilities, foodborne illness, HACCP, purchasing, receiving, storing, preparing and serving food, equipment and utensils, cleaning, sanitizing, pest control, facilities, safety and accident prevention, training, and federal and local rules and regulations. Includes illustrations, flowcharts, and a sample test.

Food Additives

American Chemical Society. *Food Flavor and Safety: Molecular Analysis and Design.* Washington, DC: American Chemical Society, 1993. 352p. ISBN 0841226652. Out of print.

This work is based on a symposium sponsored by the Division of Agricultural and Food Chemistry of the American Chemical Society to study molecular approaches to improve food quality of both plant and animal foods. A variety of topics is addressed: flavor perception and compounds affecting flavor, quality analysis, and research applications for producing quality foods, including examples from raspberries, white bread, soy sauce, and meat products. Food microbiology topics include irradiation and use of antimicrobial peptides produced by frogs, bacteria, and insects to preserve food. Each article is preceded by an abstract. Articles vary in readability; some are very technical.

Council of Europe. *Nitrates and Nitrites in Foodstuffs.* Croton-on-Hudson, NY: Manhattan Publishing, 1993. 125p. ISBN 9287124256. Out of print.

Nitrates and nitrites are widely used in the production of cured meats and to preserve fish in some countries. The additives are used to improve flavor, enhance shelf life of meat products, and protect against bacterial spoilage and hazards caused by *clostridium botulinum.* However, nitrates and nitrites can be harmful, causing mutagenic effects in in vitro systems. This report discusses the use of nitrates and nitrites and gives tables of permitted levels by country.

Davidson, P. Michael, and Alfred Branen. *Antimicrobials in Food.* New York: Marcel Dekker, 1993. 664p. ISBN 0824789067, $250.

This work covers both added and naturally occurring antimicrobials, providing detailed information about their spectrum of activity, mechanisms of action, application, regulations, toxicological aspects, and assays. A helpful introduction, a section on antibiotic residues in foods and their significance, and methods of evaluation enhance the value of this book.

Hull, Janet Starr. *Sweet Poison: How the World's Most Popular Artificial Sweetener Is Killing Us—My Story.* Fox Hills, NJ: New Horizon Press, 1999. 300p. ISBN 0882821644, $25.95.

In this first-person account, the author describes her illness and subsequent recovery after eliminating aspartame from her diet. Hull became very ill and was diagnosed with Graves disease. Before agreeing to have her thyroid removed, Hull decided to trace the cause of her illness. She determined that she was suffering from aspartame poisoning and stopped drinking diet sodas. After she got well, she researched aspartame and made contact with other sufferers. She includes case studies of other patients, gives scientific reasons aspartame can negatively react with human physiology, gives tips for staying healthy, and includes an appendix of organizations, resources, and testimony presented to Congress regarding aspartame.

Millstone, Erik. *Food Additives: Taking the Lid off What We Really Eat.* Harmondsworth, Middlesex, England: Penguin Books, 1986. 162p. Out of print.

Millstone decided to investigate food additives in Britain after reading a U.S. article that argued that the food industry in the United States was using chemical additives in ways that enabled them to enhance profitability but failed to guarantee that no harm was being done to consumers. This is a well-researched look at the economic relationship between food additives and the food business and includes information about the safety of various food additives.

Roberts, H. J. *Aspartame (NutraSweet): Is It Safe?* Philadelphia: Charles Press, 1990. 315p. ISBN 0914783378, $26.95.

Roberts, an internist with outstanding credentials, includes his personal observations of patients along with a summary of the scientific literature regarding aspartame. In 1985 over 800 million pounds were used in the United States in over 1,200 different products. Of all complaints directed to the FDA 80 percent are regarding aspartame. The licensing process is discussed as well as the physiological process aspartame can have on the body when it is metabolized. Roberts conducted original research on the subject and has found that women are three times more sensitive to aspartame than men. Symptoms of aspartame sensitivity are described and substitutes are suggested.

Schwartz, George. *In Bad Taste: The MSG Symptom Complex* 2nd ed. Santa Fe, NM: Health Press, 1999. 179p. ISBN 0929173309 (paper), $14.95.

Monosodium glutamate (MSG) is the most widely used flavor enhancer after salt and pepper. The author, a medical doctor, states that 30 percent of adults and 10–20 percent of children have some reaction to MSG. Symptoms can include asthma, acute headaches, heart irregularities, extreme mood swings, irritability, depression, rage reactions, and paranoia. Besides describing adverse reactions, the author describes the economic reasons MSG is used, gives ingredient names that can indicate the presence of MSG, and includes recipes for some of the most common sauces that contain MSG commercially.

Stoddard, Mary Nash, ed. *Deadly Deception: Story of Aspartame.* Dallas, TX: Aspartame Consumer Safety Network, 1996. ISBN 1884363148, $25.

This collection of articles has information about aspartame, the commonly used artificial sweetener found in diet soft drinks and many other products. A timeline and information about the Aspartame Consumer Safety Network and its founder, Mary Nash Stoddard, are included.

Tennant, David, ed. *Food Chemical Risk Analysis.* New York: Blackie Academic and Professional, 1997. 470p. ISBN 0412723107, $135.

The authors present new methods for analyzing the risks of food additives. Because animal studies are expensive and unpopular, other methods are being considered, including a technique where cells are treated with chemicals in laboratories, human studies using epidemiological data or volunteers, and the use of computerized molecular modeling and expert software systems to analyze hazards. Quantitative risk assessment, biomarkers in epidemiological and toxicological nutrition research, estimating dietary intake of food chemicals, assessing risks to infants and children, dietary chemoprevention in toxicological perspectives, prioritization of possible carcinogenic hazards in food, threshold of regulation, understanding the role in human health of non-nutrient chemicals in food, and risk management are also considered.

30th Meeting of the Joint FAO/WHO Expert Committee on Food Additives. *Toxicological Evaluation of Certain Food Additives and Contaminants.* New York: Cambridge University Press, 1986. 255p. Out of print.

Published on behalf of WHO, this work includes toxicological studies of antioxidants including BHA and BHT, coloring agents, the sweetening agent mannitol, thickening agents including Tara and Xanthan gums, miscellaneous food additives, and the contaminant lead. Appendixes cover reports and other documents from previous meetings of the committee, abbreviations, acceptable daily intakes, and other toxicological recommendations.

Tschanz, Christian, et al., eds. *The Clinical Evaluation of a Food Additive: Assessment of Aspartame.* Boca Raton, FL: CRC Press, 1996. 308p. ISBN 0849349737, $144.95.

Overview of various aspects of the safety evaluation process of a food additive, including a historical perspective of the development of good clinical practice guidelines and review of current regulatory requirements for conducting research on humans. Using aspartame as an example, the work shows clinical research, the types of studies needed to evaluate metabolism and pharmacokinetics of food additives in humans, how safety of additives is determined during pregnancy, and evaluation of aspartame on certain at-risk subgroups including those with liver and renal problems. One chapter evaluates the anecdotal medical complaints received from consumers of aspartame. All of the editors of this volume work for Monsanto, the developer of aspartame.

Food Safety in Commercial Applications

Bryan, Frank. *Hazard Analysis Critical Control Point Evaluations: A Guide to Identifying Hazards and Assessing Risks Associated with Food Preparation and Storage.* Geneva, Switzerland: World Health Organization, 1992. 72p. ISBN 9241544333, $12.

Taking a practical approach, this guide is designed to help public health personnel evaluate homes, cottage industries, street stalls, schools, and food service establishments where monitoring and control criteria may not lend themselves to sophisticated monitoring. These procedures emphasize the operation rather than the physical facility, which may often be less than ideal in many countries. A thorough discussion of the HACCP system, how and where to conduct an evaluation, how to analyze hazards and evaluate the severity of risks, and what toxins and bacteria to look for in various foods are included. HACCP diagrams for household food preparations of rice and infant formula are given as examples. Includes references.

Chesworth, N., ed. *Food Hygiene Auditing.* Gaithersburg, MD: Aspen Publishing, 1997. 198p. ISBN 0834216809, $100.

This work is designed to enable the reader to perform an audit of a processing facility for compliance with HACCP principles. Includes relevant food laws in the United Kingdom and United States, how the premises should be designed, how to audit raw material, processing equipment and machinery hygiene standards, preventative pest control, cleaning and disinfecting systems, and management controls.

Hemminger, Jane. *Food Safety: A Guide to What You Really Need to Know.* Ames: Iowa State University Press, 2000. 96p. ISBN 0813824826 (paper), $24.95.

This humorous guide is accessible to a range of audiences and includes HACCP guidelines, food hazards, food preparation and service, cleaning and sanitation, trash, and pests. A sanitation walk-through of all food preparation areas and recommended storage times for refrigerators, freezers, and storerooms add to the practicality of this guide. Illustrations and quizzes.

Loken, Joan. *HACCP Food Safety Manual.* New York: John Wiley and Sons, 1995. 318p. ISBN 0471056855, $69.95.

A professional HACCP trainer, Loken has designed this manual for the food service industry. Practically oriented, it includes many examples and signs that could be duplicated for use in a food service establishment. Many of the signs are written in both Spanish and English. Flowcharts, graphs, illustrations, checklists, and quizzes are used throughout to make the material easier to use. A chapter on foodborne illnesses, a glossary, and a resources section are included.

Mick, Martin, and James Budd. *Food Safety Management and Compliance.* Madison, NJ: Food Safety Institute, 1996. ISBN 0965273202, $245.

Designed to enable restaurants and other food service vendors to implement and maintain a food safety program, this loose-leaf manual covers understanding the food code, management and personnel, food, equipment, utensils, linens, water, plumbing, waste, physical facilities, compliance and enforcement, professional hygiene, handling complaints, relevance of HACCP, person in charge, foodborne illness, and future regulations. Includes an index and glossary.

Mortimore, Sara, and Carol Wallace. *HACCP: A Practical Approach,* 2nd ed. Gaithersburg, MD: Aspen Publishers, 1998. 403p. ISBN 0412754401, $69.

This very practical manual explains terms clearly, presents the theory behind HACCP rules, and uses case studies from the U.K., Ireland, Canada, South America, and Asia to illustrate how to do a HACCP study, implement the plan, and maintain the system. The authors link HACCP with other quality management techniques. Illustrations, tables, references, and resources.

Stevenson, Kenneth, and Dane Bernard. *HACCP: Establishing Hazard Analysis Critical Control Point Programs: A Workshop Manual,* 2nd ed. Washington, DC: Food Processors' Institute, 1995. 224p. ISBN 0937774030, $50.

This widely used manual was developed by the Food Processors' Institute and is based on the seven principles of HACCP as defined by the National Advisory Committee on Microbiological Criteria for Foods. Not specific to any product category, it is general enough to be used as a step-by-step guide for establishing a HACCP program for any food product.

United States Department of Agriculture. *List of Proprietary Substances and Non-Food Compounds Authorized for Use under USDA Inspections and Grading Programs.* Washington, DC: U.S. Government Printing Office. Published annually.

This publication lists all substances that have been approved and authorized by the Food Safety and Inspection Service (FSIS) for use in agricultural production. The list is organized alphabetically by trade name under the heading of the firm by which it is marketed.

Food Safety Law and Policy

Antle, John M. *Choice and Efficiency in Food Safety Policy.* Washington, DC: AEI Press, 1995. 105p. ISBN 0844739022 (case), $29.95; ISBN 0844739030 (paper), $14.95.

This work, sponsored by the American Enterprise Institute, looks at food safety policy from an economic point of view. The author, an agricultural economist, examines conditions under which food safety regulation is needed, what kinds of changes in existing legislation could move the current system toward safer food at a lower cost, and considers what role farm bill legislation should play in achieving food safety policy goals. As an example, Antle believes too much attention is placed on pesticide regulation at the expense of foodborne disease prevention and diseases associated with diet.

Arnold, Andrea. *Fear of Food: Environmentalist Scams, Media Mendacity, and the Law of Disparagement.* Bellevue, WA: Free Enterprise Press, 1990. 155p. ISBN 0939571080, $9.95.

Arnold gives a history of the pesticide Alar and claims that the Natural Resources Defense Council manipulated the media into sensationalist treatment of the pesticide in order to gain subscribers for their organization. Alar was banned by the EPA in 1989.

Institute of Medicine, National Research Council. *Ensuring Safe Food: From Production to Consumption.* Washington, DC: National Academy Press, 1998. 194p. ISBN 0309065593, $19.95.

At the request of the United States Congress, the Agricultural Research Service of the United States Department of Agriculture asked the National Academy of Sciences in 1997 to determine the scientific basis of an effective food safety system. This is the report of the academy's conclusions regarding the effectiveness of the current food safety system in the United States, scientific needs and gaps within the current system, and recommendations on scientific and organizational changes in federal food safety activity needed to ensure an effective, science-based food safety system.

Powell, Douglas, and William Leiss. *Mad Cows and Mother's Milk: The Perils of Poor Risk Communication.* Toronto: McGill Queens University Press, 1997. 336p. ISBN 0773516900, $19.95.

Using a case study approach, the authors discuss the problem of communicating health risks without creating undue public fear. Risk management strategies are presented for communicating the nature and consequences of environmental and health risks to the public.

Schumann, Michael, et al. *Food Safety Law.* New York: Van Nostrand Reinhold, 1997. 325p. ISBN 0442022166, $69.95.

This helpful work describes the different branches of U.S. government involved with food safety and the regulatory and legal authority each has. A food sanitation manual is included in an appendix. The Humane Slaughter Act, Poultry Products Inspection Act, descriptions of foodborne illnesses, descriptions of HACCP, descriptions of how to manage facility safety and sanitation programs, and selected cases are included.

Foodborne Diseases

Eley, Adrian. *Microbial Food Poisoning,* 2nd ed. New York: Chapman and Hall, 1996. 211p. ISBN 0412644304. (Note: This summary refers to the second edition, which is now out of print. The third edition is in press at this writing and has the following publication information: Eley, Adrian. *Microbial Food Poisoning,* 3rd ed. New York: Chapman and Hall, 2000. 240p. ISBN 0412373904, $49.50.)

Discusses infective bacterial causes of foodborne illness such as salmonella and campylobacter, toxic bacterial causes such as staphylococcus and clostridium, other bacterial pathogens like listeria, and mycotoxic fungi, viruses, and protozoa. Also includes lab diagnosis, epidemiology, trends in food poisoning, factors contributing to food poisoning, food industry notification and reporting, investigation, surveillance and epidemiology of specific organisms, microbiological control of food production, food safety, food legislation, and food hygiene. Laws mentioned pertain to the United Kingdom where this book was first published.

Fox, Nicols. *Spoiled: The Dangerous Truth about a Food Chain Gone Haywire.* New York: Basic Books, 1997. 434p. ISBN 0465019803 (case), $25; ISBN 014027555X (paper), $14.95.

The author, a journalist, details the changing nature of foodborne disease, giving accounts of particular incidents including *E. coli* outbreaks from apple juice and hamburger, salmonella, mad cow disease, and campylobacter, a bacteria that affects chickens. Each pathogen is carefully explained, causes of contamination are explored, and the response of public health officials is reported. The author argues that globalization of food sources and increased food processing have increased the amount and severity of foodborne illness at a time when spending on public health has declined. A final chapter discusses safe food practices from a consumer viewpoint.

Heersink, Mary. *E. Coli O157:H7: The True Story of a Mother's Battle with a Killer Microbe.* Far Hills, NJ: New Horizon Press, 1996. 303p. ISBN 0882821431, $22.95.

In 1992 Mary Heersink's son, Damion, ate some undercooked hamburger on a Boy Scouts outing and developed severe food poisoning from *E. coli* O157:H7. Damion Heersink developed hemolytic uremic syndrome, an often fatal condition that can permanently damage the heart, kidneys, and other organs. Heersink recounts the course of her son's illness in diary format including her investigation into the cause of the illness. A helpful afterword by Carol Tucker Foreman of the Safe Food Coalition gives statistics about *E. coli* and foodborne illness and describes the legislative efforts of Safe Tables Our Priority, the organization Mary Heersink helped found after her son's poisoning.

Hui, Y. H. J., Richard Gorham, K. D. Murrell, and Dean Cliver, eds. *Foodborne Disease Handbook.* New York: Marcel Dekker, 1994. 3 volumes. Volume 1: ISBN 0824790634, Volume 2: ISBN 0824791657, Volume 3: ISBN 0824791665, $189 per volume.

Volume 1, *Diseases Caused by Bacteria,* has chapters on bacterial diseases as well as surveillance of foodborne disease, indicator organisms in food, and investigating foodborne disease. Volume

2 covers viruses, parasites, and fungal toxins transmitted via food. General topics in this volume include information on epidemiology, clinical aspects of foodborne disease, laboratory methods for diagnosis, and causative agents. Volume 3, *Diseases Caused by Hazardous Substances,* covers naturally occurring chemicals in food, poisonous plants, toxic marine mammals, drug residues in foods of animal origin, radioactivity in food and water, toxicology and risk assessment, hard foreign objects in food as a cause of injury, and food, filth, and disease. Each article contains many references, and each volume has an index.

Rampton, Sheldon, and John Stauber. *Mad Cow U.S.A.: Could the Nightmare Happen Here?* Monroe, ME: Common Courage Press, 1997. 224p. ISBN 1567511112, $24.95.

The authors argue that both the U.S. and British governments colluded with beef producers to suppress important facts about interspecies transmission of bovine spongiform encephalopathy (BSE), and that it would be quite possible for a mad cow–type situation to happen in the United States. They also discuss the food disparagement laws and how these laws have made it harder for people to question food safety publicly, when even the media get sued for tackling safety issues.

Ratzan, Scott, ed. *The Mad Cow Crisis: Health and the Public Good.* New York: New York University Press, 1998. 247p. ISBN 0814775101 (case), $55; ISBN 081477511X (paper), $18.50.

Using a multidisciplinary approach, Ratzan has gathered viewpoints from experts across a variety of fields. Includes effective communication of health and risk issues, veterinary history of the disease, a history of transmissible spongiform encephalopathies, a discussion of whether the spread of BSE and CJD is predictable, decision theory as it relates to BSE communications, political and public health considerations, media coverage on BSE in Britain and the United States, avoiding crises in the future, farming with nature, and strategies for obtaining public health.

Rhodes, Richard. *Deadly Feasts: Tracking the Secrets of a Terrifying New Plague.* New York: Simon and Schuster, 1997. 259p. ISBN 0684823608, $24.

Starting with kuru, the transmissible spongiform encephalopathy (TSE) found among cannibals in the Fore tribe in New

Guinea, this book traces TSEs from scrapie in sheep, to an unnamed TSE in mink, to bovine spongiform encephalopathy (BSE), to new variant Creutzfeldt-Jakob disease (nvCJD). Rhodes concludes that BSE is in the United States in native form (it occurs spontaneously at a rate of 1:1,000,000). Through cannibalism, which occurs with ruminant-to-ruminant feeding, it could be intensified and occur at a higher rate. The handling of BSE in Britain is discussed, and the author believes that the government failed to provide adequate inspection, supervision, and policy to mitigate the crisis. The U.S. ban on ruminant-to-ruminant feeding is too watered down to prevent the passage of TSEs between species in the author's view.

Steele, John, ed. *Clinics in Laboratory Diseases: Food Borne Diseases* 19, no. 3 (September 1999). 712p. ISSN 02722712.

This work is a thorough review of most of the causes of foodborne illness. Each article discusses the microbiological and toxicological features of the pathogen and describes the disease, including pathogenesis, epidemiology, and clinical features. Geared toward medical professionals, this work gives diagnostic approaches for labs, physician offices, and field studies as well as therapeutic options and ideas for prevention.

General

Bronner, Felix, ed. *Nutrition Policy in Public Health.* New York: Springer Publishing, 1997. 363p. ISBN 0826196608, $52.95.

This work covers policy regarding many food issues, including nutrition-related conditions and diseases such as inadequate nutrition, obesity, heart disease, dental caries prevention, and at-risk populations. Two very helpful chapters cover foodborne diseases and the legal aspects of food protection. Includes information on food additives, pesticides, and microbes, as well as regulatory information about the United States.

Jones, Julie Miller. *Food Safety.* St. Paul, MN: Eagan Press, 1992. ISBN 0962440736, $99.

This textbook of food safety includes a history of food laws, how risk-benefit analysis is used in food safety determinations, naturally occurring toxicants, bacteriological problems, molds, mycotoxins, parasites, viruses, effects of food processing, food additives, colors, flavors, irradiation, pesticides, incidental contaminants, and radionuclides in food.

McCuen, Gary, ed. *Poison in Your Food.* Ideas in Conflict Series. Hudson, WI: Gary E. McCuen Publications, 1991. 160p. ISBN 086596078X, $12.95.

This collection contains articles on both sides of the food safety debate, including pro and con articles about organic produce, seafood safety, food irradiation, pesticides, dioxin, and meat. A bibliography, cartoons, and questions for study are included.

Millichap, J. Gordon. *Environmental Poisons in Our Food.* Chicago, IL: PNB Publishers, 1993. 271p. ISBN 0962911577, $14.95.

Each of the fourteen chapters covers a different type of food poison, including lead, trace metals, pesticide and insecticide residues, foodborne and waterborne infections and toxins, food additives, excess vitamin toxicity, alcohol and caffeine, and food allergies. A final chapter describes food safety controls. Each chapter is well laid out and describes symptoms, prevention, incidence, sources of the poison, treatment, and prognosis. Although written by a pediatric neurologist, the work is easily understood by the lay reader.

University of the Netherlands. *Food Safety and Toxicity.* Boca Raton, FL: CRC Press, 1997. 349p. ISBN 0849394880, $74.95.

Traces food from raw material to processing, preparation, choices made by the consumer, to physiological effect on the body. The effect of dietary behavior (e.g., dieting, overeating, and undereating) on food choice is considered, along with how changes in dietary behavior influence risk management. Emphasis is on toxicological risks rather than microbial ones. Although there is a lot of technical information, the writing is extremely clear. References throughout.

Van der Heijden, Kees. *International Food Safety Handbook.* New York: Marcel Dekker, 1999. 811p. ISBN 0824793544, $195.

Emphasizes the interrelationship between science, regulation, and control of food safety, even though they are often considered separately by individuals and agencies. Microbiology and hygiene aspects, drinking water safety, safety aspects of soft drinks, food additives, mycotoxins, novel foods, accidents affecting food and food poisoning, bovine spongiform encephalopathy and new variant Creutzfeldt-Jakob disease, food labeling regulations in the United States and Europe, and the shifts in food safety perception by consumers and consumer organizations are considered along with international trade issues.

Waltner-Toews, David. *Food, Sex, and Salmonella: The Risks of Environmental Intimacy.* Toronto: NC Press, 1992. Out of print.

An interesting look at food risks. The author, a veterinarian, likens eating to sex, as an act of intimacy with the environment. He recommends that we be less promiscuous in our eating habits, paying attention to where our food comes from, and choosing not to get food from certain places and sources. Includes a very good description of risk assessment.

Genetically Modified Foods

Engel, Karl-Heinz, Gary Takeoka, and Roy Teranishi, eds. *Genetically Modified Foods: Safety Issues.* Washington, DC: American Chemical Society, 1995. ISBN 0841233209, $78.95.

This volume is a result of a symposium sponsored by the American Chemical Society on the safety of genetically modified foods. Includes an introduction to what is meant by genetically modified foods; regulatory oversight in the United States, Japan, and the European Union; the role of public and federal advisory committees in the United States; safety assessment of flavor ingredients produced by genetic modifications; comparison of traditional genetic techniques (e.g., cross-breeding) with biotechnology; potential for allergic reactions to transgenic foods (e.g., nonnut foods that take properties from nuts can be a real hazard); genetic modifications to farm animals; and use of plant virus genes to produce disease-resistant crops. Abstracts precede each article.

Hopkins, D. Douglas, Rebecca Goldburg, and Steven Hirsch. *A Mutable Feast: Assuring Food Safety in the Era of Genetic Engineering/A Proposal to the FDA to Adopt New Safety and*

Labeling Rules for Genetically Engineered Foods. New York: Environmental Defense Fund, 1991. 74p.

Although this report was written in 1991, the FDA still hasn't adopted stringent requirements for genetically engineered food. This report proposes adding three rules to current FDA policy. (1) The FDA should subject new substances in genetically engineered organisms used for food to the premarket safety testing requirements for food additives. (2) Foods that contain substances from genetic engineering should be disclosed on labels. (3) There should be premarket certification by the FDA in the composition of all genetically engineered whole foods.

Organization for Economic Cooperation and Development (OECD). *Aquatic Biotechnology and Food Safety.* Washington, DC: OECD Publications and Information Center, 1994. ISBN 9264140638, $18.

This publication is the proceedings of the Symposium on Aquatic Biotechnology and Food Safety held in Bergen, Norway, in June 1992. The purpose of the conference was to identify food safety implications unique to modern aquatic biotechnology. Participants from Norway, the United Kingdom, Japan, and the United States contributed to the conference.

Organization for Economic Cooperation and Development (OECD). *Food Safety Evaluation.* Washington, DC: OECD Publications and Information Center, 1996. 180p. ISBN 9264148671, $36.

This work is the result of a workshop designed to explore strategies for evaluating the safety of biotechnology when there are no acceptable counterparts for comparison. Test procedures for bioengineered tomatoes and squash are described. The transgenic, insect-resistant Bt tomato attacks the digestive systems of insects. Feeding studies with rats given the equivalent of 500 to 2,000 kilograms of the tomatoes showed no ill effects.

Organization for Economic Cooperation and Development. *Safety Evaluation of Foods Derived by Modern Biotechnology: Concepts and Principles.* Paris: Organization for Economic Cooperation and Development, 1993. 79p. ISBN 9264138595. Out of print.

This report is based on work done by the Group of National Experts on Safety in Biotechnology. The group found that the most practical way to determine the safety of foods produced by biotechnology is to consider whether the products are substantially equivalent to analogous conventional food products, if they exist. Products are compared on the basis of nutritive value, toxicants, dietary exposure, and other relevant factors. Several case studies show how particular foods can be evaluated.

History

Coppin, Clayton, and Jack High. *Politics of Purity: Harvey Washington Wiley and the Origins of Federal Food Policy.* Ann Arbor, MI: University of Michigan Press, 1999. 219p. ISBN 0472109847, $49.50.

The authors examine the economics and politics behind the 1906 pure food law. They conclude that Harvey Wiley, the principal regulator behind the pure food laws, acted to nationalize regulation in order to concentrate his own power, and his actions gave competitive advantage to national brands over local ones. Uniform national labels and regulations favored national brands that could prepare food and label it to one standard rather than having to make separate labels for each state. The authors argue that the national food concerns supported national food legislation because it was a strategic use of public policy.

Goodwin, Lorine. *Pure Food and Drink Crusaders, 1879–1914.* Jefferson, NC: McFarland, 1999. 352p. ISBN 0786406186, $45.

Goodwin discusses the individual women and women's groups who became concerned about the food, drink, and drugs that were affecting their families, and what they did about it. The author argues that the crusaders were instrumental in mobilizing government to enact pure food laws, and that without consumer pressure, the laws would not have been enacted.

Whorton, James. *Before Silent Spring: Pesticides and Public Health in Pre-DDT America.* Princeton, NJ: Princeton University Press, 1974. 288p. ISBN 0691081395. Out of print.

Whorton traces the use of chemical pesticides since their introduction in the 1860s, tracking the origins of the residue problem and exploring the interest groups that formed around the issue, including how economic necessities, technological limitations, and pressures on regulatory agencies have brought us to our current high level of pesticide use.

Wiley, Harvey. *Foods and Their Adulteration.* Philadelphia: P. P. Blakiston's and Sons, 1907. 625p. Out of print.

This classic gives the origin, manufacture, and composition of foods. Descriptions of common adulterations, food standards, and national food laws and regulations. Much of the information is still useful, but some has historical interest only.

Young, James Harvey. *Pure Food: Securing the Federal Food and Drug Act of 1906.* Princeton, NJ: Princeton University Press, 1989. 312p. ISBN 0691047634. Out of print.

Young, a historian, examines the sixty years that preceded the Pure Food Bill to show the various factors and people that made the law come about. The work includes discussion of the adulteration of drugs used during the Mexican-American War, mercury poisoning, adulterated meat and milk, glucose and oleo margarine, the impact of technology, political history of the law, the effect of Upton Sinclair's *The Jungle,* and how the law, after it finally passed, was interpreted.

Irradiation and Other Methods of Preservation

Cassens, Robert. *Meat Preservation: Preventing Losses and Assuring Safety.* Trumbull, CT: Food and Nutrition Press, 1994. 133p. ISBN 0917678346, $72.

Cassens provides both a historical and current look at meat preservation. Includes historical aspects and trends, basic background information, evolution and status of techniques and procedures, and potential future developments. Chapters highlight how to understand muscle and meat; the meat industry; the goals of preservation; the physical, chemical, and microbial methods of preservation; and how to manage preservation. Cassens notes that military and exploration efforts drove new technology in meat preservation in the past, while today preservation is primarily consumer driven.

Diehl, J. F. *Safety of Irradiated Foods,* 2nd ed. New York: Marcel Dekker, 1995. 454p. ISBN 0824793447, $189.

History of irradiation; radiation sources; chemical effects of ionizing radiation; biological effects; identification of irradiated foods; radiological, toxicological, and microbiological safety of irradiated foods; nutritional adequacy of irradiated foods; evaluation of wholesomeness; potential and current applications; government regulations; and consumer attitudes are all included in this comprehensive work on irradiation. An appendix contains the Codex standards for irradiated foods and a glossary of terms.

Gould, G. W., ed. *New Methods of Food Preservation.* New York: Blackie Academic and Professional, 1995. 324p. ISBN 0751400483, $93.

This technical work covers major trends in food processing: applications of modified atmosphere packaging (MAP); use of naturally occurring antimicrobials including animal-, plant-, and microorganism-derived substances; ways to deliver heat to foods; high hydrostatic pressures to inactivate microorganisms; high-voltage electric pulses; ultrasonic radiation for pasteurization and sterilization; and food surface decontamination procedures.

Murray, David. *Biology of Food Irradiation.* New York: John Wiley and Sons, 1990. 255p. ISBN 0471926213, $139.

A biologist discusses the disadvantages of irradiation. Includes information about electron spin resonance techniques that would allow irradiated food to be identified, making it feasible to enforce bans on irradiation.

Satin, Morton. *Food Irradiation: A Guidebook.* Lancaster, PA: Technomic Publishing, 1996. ISBN 1566763444, $62.95.

The author, the director of Agricultural Services for the Food and Agriculture Organization of the UN, argues that irradiation is safe, and that the struggle to adopt it is similar to consumers' previous reluctance to embrace pasteurization of milk. This work is aimed at consumers and provides plenty of nontechnical information.

VanGarde, Shirley, and Margy Woodburn. *Food Preservation and Safety: Principles and Practices.* Ames: Iowa State University, 1994. ISBN 0813821339, $42.95.

Explains how to preserve foods and why specific processes and safety precautions are beneficial or necessary.

Microbiology of Foods

Garbutt, John. *Essentials of Food Microbiology.* New York: Oxford University Press, 1997. 251p. ISBN 0340677015, $34.50.

Food microbiology is the study of the role that microorganisms play in food spoilage, food production, food preservation, and foodborne disease. The author, an instructor in food microbiology, assumes no previous knowledge of microbiology and explains microbiological principles in the context of food.

Topics include structure of microorganisms, naming, classification, and identification of microorganisms, growth of microorganisms and microbial populations, microbial nutrition and cultivation, factors affecting growth, death of microorganisms and microbial populations, food spoilage, foodborne disease and food poisoning, fermented foods, and controlling microbiological quality and safety of foods.

Roberts, T. A., A. C. Baird-Parker, R. B. Tompkin, eds. *Microorganisms in Food 5: Characteristics of Microbial Pathogens.* New York: Chapman and Hall, 1996. 513p. ISBN 041247350X. Out of print.

Organized by name of microorganism, each entry features history, taxonomy, symptoms, pathogenicity, detection and enumeration, identification, distribution in nature and importance in food, problem in foods, factors affecting growth, factors affecting inhibition, death, survival, toxic characteristics, and production control. Tables and references. This is the fifth title in the series published by the International Commission on Microbial Specifications for foods. The other volumes in the series are subtitled *Their Significance and Methods of Enumeration, Sampling for Microbial Analysis: Principles and Specific Applications, Microbial Ecology of Foods: Factors Affecting Growth and Death of Microorganism* (Volume 1), *Microbial Ecology of Foods: Food*

Commodities (Volume 2), and *Application of Hazard Analysis (HACCP) System to Ensure Microbial Safety and Quality.*

Vanderzant, Carl, and Don Splittstoesser. *Compendium of Methods for the Microbiological Examination of Foods,* 3rd ed. Washington, DC: American Public Health Association, 1992. 1,219p. ISBN 0875531733, $90.

General lab procedures, quality assurance, sampling plans, and sample collection are explained. Microbiological monitoring of the food processing environment, microorganisms involved in the processing and spoilage of food, indicator microorganisms and pathogens including most bacteria that cause foodborne illness, and rapid and/or automatic methods for microbial examination are included as well as how to investigate foodborne illness outbreaks and how to deal with viruses, parasites, and toxins.

Pesticides

Mott, Laurie, and Karen Snyder. *Pesticide Alert: A Guide to Pesticides in Fruits and Vegetables.* San Francisco: Sierra Club Books, 1987. ISBN 0871567288 (case), ISBN 0871567261 (paper). Out of print.

Discusses the dangers of pesticides. The majority of the book is an alphabetical summary of produce items, with what pesticides are used on each produce item and how to reduce risks. Contains tables, a glossary, and a bibliography organized by pesticide name.

National Research Council. *Pesticides in the Diets of Infants and Children.* Washington, DC: National Academy Press, 1993. 386p. ISBN 0309048753, $47.95.

In 1988 Congress requested the National Academy of Sciences to study the scientific and policy issues concerning pesticides in the diets of infants and children. The committee found both quantitative and sometimes qualitative differences in toxicity of pesticides between children and adults. Qualitative differences are consequences of exposure during certain windows of vulnerability. The committee recommended that changes be made to the way pesticides were regulated so that the estimates of expected

total exposure to pesticide residues reflect the unique characteristics of the diets of infants and children and include the nondi-
etary intake of pesticides from landscaping, etc. (Partly as a result
of this study, the Food Quality Protection Act of 1996 was enacted. The new law requires that all exposures to pesticides must
be shown to be safe for infants and children.)

Steinman, David. *Diet for a Poisoned Planet.* New York:
Harmony Books, 1990. 392p. ISBN 0517575124 (case), $21.95;
ISBN 0517104113 (paper), $3.99.

Using the FDA's total diet study data to determine what foods
have the lowest concentrations of pesticides, the author divided
each food group into green light, yellow light, and red light
foods. He advocates a plant-based diet because plant foods are
lowest in pesticides. (Pesticides bioaccumulate in animal products. As an animal eats grains grown with pesticides, the pesticides persist in the animal's body, accumulating to levels much
higher than in plant foods.) Lists tell which pesticides are associated with each food and an appendix gives detailed information
about particular pesticides.

Wargo, John. *Our Children's Toxic Legacy: How Science and Law
Fail to Protect Us from Pesticides.* New Haven, CT: Yale
University Press, 1996. 380p. ISBN 0300066864 (case), $35; ISBN
0300074468 (paper), $18.

Wargo traces pesticide use and regulation from the mid-twentieth
century to the 1990s. His analysis shows that public and expert
views of pesticides focused on short-term benefits. Gradually
key laws and regulations followed the evolving understanding
of pesticide-related risks. The author concludes that the EPA's
inconsistent application of the risk-balancing standard of the
Federal Insecticide, Fungicide, and Rodenticide Act (FIFRA) was
responsible for the vast majority of pesticide-related cancer risk
in the American diet. He believes that science and pesticide law
has distracted government agencies and the public from identifying and managing significant risks and includes some suggestions for reform.

Weir, David, and Mark Schapiro. *Circle of Poison.* San Francisco:
Institute for Food and Development Policy, 1981. 99p. ISBN
0935028099. Out of print.

According to the World Health Organization, someone in a less developed nation is poisoned by pesticides every minute. Many of these pesticides are banned in the United States, but manufactured here and shipped overseas. Besides the damage to native populations, many of these same pesticides return to the United States in the form of pesticide residues on imported produce. The FDA does check produce coming into the United States, but it only tests for 30 percent of known illegal pesticides. This work, though written many years ago, documents a situation continuing today despite legislative attempts to stop it.

Winston, Mark. *Nature Wars: People vs. Pests.* Cambridge, MA: Harvard University Press, 1997. 210p. ISBN 0674605411 (case), $24.95; ISBN 067460542X (paper), $15.95.

An entomologist discusses the attitudes that lead people to choose chemical pesticides over biological controls. The author contends that humans consider themselves as separate from and more important than the rest of life. Because we treat the earth with an attitude of dominion rather than stewardship, we choose cheaper but more environmentally destructive chemical means of controlling insects instead of less harmful but more expensive biological controls. Several insect-control case studies from the United States and Canada are presented.

Winter, Carl, James Seiber, and Carole Nuckton, eds. *Chemicals in the Human Food Chain.* New York: Van Nostrand Reinhold, 1990. 276p. ISBN 0442004214, $49.95.

This work reports the findings of the University of California Agricultural Issues Center study of chemicals in the human food chain conducted in 1987–1988. The group included experts from UC Berkeley, Davis, and Riverside, and from Stanford University in the areas of veterinary medicine, medical and health sciences, nutrition, environmental toxicology, agricultural economics, food science, agronomy, pomology, and entomology. They studied five major sources of chemicals in the human food chain, including pesticides, animal products, food additives, industrial and environmental chemicals, and natural toxins. The general conclusion is that these chemicals don't cause substantial problems and are economically necessary.

Toxins and Contaminants

Boyd, Eldon. *Toxicity of Pure Foods.* Boca Raton, FL: CRC Press, 1973. 263p. ISBN 087819035X, $56.

This book describes animal studies done to determine lethal doses of pure foods such as sucrose, starch, proteins, water, salts, natural food toxicants, and caffeine.

Boyd, Eldon. *Predictive Toxicometrics.* Bristol, U.K.: Scientechnica, 1972. 408p. ISBN 0856080024. Out of print.

Predictive toxicometrics is the discipline of predicting toxic reactions and the safety of chemical agents in the general population from samples of the same or similar populations. Generally, animal studies are used to determine toxicity for humans. Although this work is quite technical, it explains the process and gives examples of calculating toxicity for certain food additives and foodborne pathogens.

Chen, Edwin. *PBB: An American Tragedy.* Englewood Cliffs, NJ: Prentice Hall, 1979. 329p. ISBN 0136546080. Out of print.

In 1973 a mix-up at a chemical company resulted in approximately one ton of the dangerous chemical polybrominated biphenyl (PBB) being mixed into dairy cattle feed in Michigan. By the time the source was located, most farm animals and virtually the entire human population of Michigan were exposed to the chemical. Chen's focus is on the slow and inadequate response of government to the crisis.

Council of Europe. *Lead, Cadmium, and Mercury in Food: Assessment of Dietary Intakes and Summary of Heavy Metal Limits of Foodstuffs.* Croton-on-Hudson, NY: Manhattan Publishing, 1994. 59p. ISBN 9287126208, $12.

Lead has been limited since as early as 1925 in some countries, mercury began being limited in the 1970s, and cadmium in the early 1980s. This thorough treatment of limits describes how limits are set and gives tables of values; factors affecting limit setting; information about how data are collected, including duplicate diet studies, total diet studies, and diaries; and the treatment of nonstandard consumers (consumers who suffer from certain medical conditions or eat unusual diets). Some European countries set limits for all products, others set limits on a particular set of foodstuffs. The legal ramifications of limits are also discussed. including those that have the force of law and those that trigger further investigation.

Eaton, David, and John Groopman, eds. *Toxicology of Aflatoxins: Human Health, Veterinary and Agricultural Significance.* San Diego: Academic Press, 1994. 544p. ISBN 0122282558, $73.

Aflatoxins are natural fungal toxins found in foods and animal feeds. The chemistry, biochemistry, toxicology, and epidemiology of aflatoxins are better understood than any other environmentally occurring chemical carcinogen. The contributors to this volume present the basic and applied toxicology of aflatoxins, including analytical identification, agricultural and veterinary implications, toxicology and carcinogenesis in humans, and economic and regulatory problems associated with aflatoxin contaminant control.

Eggington, Joyce. *Poisoning of Michigan.* New York: W. W. Norton, 1980. 351p. ISBN 0393013472. Out of print.

In 1973, a Michigan truck driver delivered a ton of what was thought to be magnesium oxide, a crumbly white substance mixed into dairy feed to help cows' digestion, to Farm Bureau Services, the operator of the largest agricultural feed plant in Michigan. A mistake had been made at the chemical factory and a similar substance, the fire retardant crystallized polybrominated biphenyl (PBB), was added to several large batches of cattle feed. Tens of thousands of farm animals became deathly ill, milk production fell, many calves died, lambs were born with gross deformities, and virtually everyone in Michigan consumed contaminated meat and dairy products before the mistake was caught. Eggington chronicles the contamination, the fortunate detective work of the farmer who discovered the problem, and the legal, political, and health consequences to the people of Michigan.

Moffat, Colin, and Kevin Whittle, eds. *Environmental Contaminants in Food.* Boca Raton, FL: CRC Press, 1999. 584p. ISBN 0849397359, $139.95.

The scope of this work includes major substances not intentionally added to food but that can be found in food as a result of general and local environmental conditions. These contaminants are radioactivity from nuclear accidents and large-scale releases from industrial and military plants, inorganic and chemical contaminants, and veterinary and pesticide residues. A chapter on safety standards for food contaminants includes estimates of consumption of particular contaminants, but the authors note the difficult nature of assessing the dangers of contaminants that might be subtle or increase cancer risk without causing illness immediately.

United States Government, Food and Drug Administration, Center for Food Safety and Applied Nutrition. *Food Defect Action Levels: Levels of Natural or Unavoidable Defects in Foods That Present No Health Hazards for Humans.* Washington, DC: U.S. Department of Health and Human Services, Public Health Service, 1994. 24p.

This work is organized by food type and gives defect, action levels at which the food must be removed from the market, the source, and significance. For example, currants may suffer from insect filth (defect). If 5 percent or more by count are wormy in the average of the subsamples (action level), the currants cannot be sold. The source of the defect is preharvest insect infestation and the significance of the infestations is aesthetic. Includes a glossary.

Selected Journals and Periodicals

Association of Food and Drug Officials Journal
Association of Food and Drug Officials
P.O. Box 3425
York, PA 17402

A refereed journal that promotes uniformity of laws affecting foods, drugs, cosmetics, devices, and product safety.

Consumer Reports
Consumers Union
101 Truman Avenue
Yonkers, NY 10703

Although this magazine covers a variety of consumer goods, food safety is an area that gets regular coverage.

FDA Consumer
U.S. Food and Drug Administration
Office of Public Affairs
5600 Fishers Lane
Rockville, MD 20857

Designed to keep the public informed about the activities of the FDA, this is a great source of information about food safety issues.

Food and Chemical Toxicology
Elsevier Science
655 Avenue of the Americas
New York, NY 10010

A refereed journal on the metabolic toxicology of foods, food, and food additives as well as carcinogens, mutagens, and drug-nutrient information.

Food and Environmental Protection Newsletter
International Atomic Energy Agency
Wagramerstrasser 5
P.O. Box 100 A-1400
Vienna, Austria

Newsletter about food irradiation. Subscriptions are free.

Food Chemical News
1725 K Street NW, Suite 506
Washington, DC 20006

This trade publication provides current information about government regulation of food and food additives.

Foodborne and Waterborne Diseases in Canada
Polyscience Publications, Inc.
P.O. Box 1606
Stn. St. Martin
Laval, PQ H7V 3P8
Canada

Summarizes information on foodborne and waterborne diseases from federal, provisional, and regional agencies in Canada.

International Food Safety News
Research Information Ltd.
222 Maylands Avenue
Hemel Hempstead, Hertsferdshire, UK HP2 7TD

A newsletter with current international news on food pathogens and food safety for public health labs, hospitals, environmental health officers, and food industry professionals.

Journal of Food Protection
International Association for Food Protection
6200 Aurora Avenue, Suite 200W
Des Moines, IA 50322

A refereed journal about food microbiology directed toward food safety professionals.

Journal of Food Safety
Food and Nutrition Press
6527 Main Street
P.O. Box 374
Trumbull, CT 06611

This technical journal presents chemical and microbiological coverage of food safety, including the toxicology, metabolism, and environmental conversion of materials entering the food supply.

Morbidity and Mortality Weekly Report
U.S. Centers for Disease Control and Prevention
1600 Clifton Road NE
Atlanta, GA 30333
Also available online for free at http://www.cdc.gov/mmwr.

This periodical is the best way to keep abreast of current foodborne disease outbreaks, pathogens, and studies about foodborne disease.

Nutrition Action Healthletter
Center for Science in the Public Interest
1875 Connecticut Avenue NW, Suite 300
Washington, DC 20009

One of the best publications oriented toward consumers about nutrition, food policy, and food safety issues.

Pesticide and Toxic Chemical News
Food Chemical News
1725 K Street NW, Suite 506
Washington, DC 20006

A loose-leaf service that keeps subscribers up-to-date on tolerances, administrative guidelines, and exemptions for pesticide residues in food and feed. Other sections cover toxic chemicals and hazardous wastes.

7

Nonprint Resources

Databases

Most libraries subscribe to computerized periodical databases either on CD-ROM or on the Internet. General databases provide access to many articles on food safety that are mostly appropriate for a general audience. For more focused searches, consult one of the technical databases listed below. Ask a librarian about access to these databases. A wide range of information can also be found on the free Internet databases listed below, and on the websites listed in Chapter 5, Directory of Organizations.

General Databases

Academic Abstracts
Ebsco
P.O. Box 92901
Los Angeles, CA 90009
(800) 683-2726

This database is available in many academic libraries. Full text is available back to 1990, and indexing and abstracting go back as far as 1984.

InfoTrac
Gale Group
P.O. Box 9187
Farmington Hills, MI 48333
(800) 877-GALE

Many public libraries offer access to InfoTrac. It has an easy-to-use interface.

Lexis Nexis
P.O. Box 933
Dayton, OH 45401
(800) 227-9597

Although originally designed for legal and business applications, many food safety topics are included in its outstanding news coverage.

ProQuest Direct
Bell and Howell
300 N. Zeeb Road
P.O. Box 1346
Ann Arbor, MI 48106
(800) 521-0600

This database is available in many academic libraries. It can be used to search magazine and newspaper articles. Organized into modules, it is possible to search in subject-specific areas like business magazines or national newspapers. The entire database can also be searched.

Specialized Databases

Agricola
Dialog
11000 Regency Parkway, Suite 10
Cary, NC 27511
(919) 462-8600

The National Agricultural Library's database has over 3.6 million citations on a variety of agricultural subjects. Materials date from 1970. (Also available from Ebsco and Gale Group.)

Food Science and Technology Abstracts
SilverPlatter
100 River Ridge Drive
Norwood, MA 02062
(800) 343-0064

Includes comprehensive coverage of research and new development literature in food science and technology. Eighty percent of the material comes from over 1,800 journals in ninety countries. The remaining material comes from patents, reviews, poster presentations, abstracts of theses, technical sessions, reports, and books. (Also available from Dialog.)

Foodline: Current Food Legislation
Dialog
11000 Regency Parkway, Suite 10
Cary, NC 27511
(919) 462-8600

Designed to give current food additive, composition, and labeling legislation. Details of permitted uses for food additives worldwide are available, as well as standards documents regarding composition and labeling requirements for seven European Union countries and the United States with product definitions and permitted ingredients.

Foodline: Science and Technology
Dialog
11000 Regency Parkway, Suite 10
Cary, NC 27511
(919) 462-8600

Abstracts of journal articles cover all aspects of the food and drink industry, including ingredients and process technology, microbiology, packaging, food chemistry, biotechnology, food safety, and nutrition.

Nutrition Abstracts and Reviews
CABI Publishing
10 E. 40th Street, Suite 3203
New York, NY 10016
(212) 481-7018

Food contamination and toxicology, pesticide and chemical residues, naturally occurring toxic substances, functional foods, food policy, food legislation, and additives are included as well as many other nutrition topics.

Pesticide Fact File
Dialog
11000 Regency Parkway, Suite 10
Cary, NC 27511
(919) 462-8600

Scientific data on component chemicals and biological active ingredients used in agrochemical formulations worldwide.

Free Internet Databases

Institute of Food Science and Technology
Website: http://www.ift.org

This is one of the best websites for food safety research. A food headlines section contains summaries of current food-related news stories, and an information gateway provides links to over 2,000 websites on a variety of topics. Best of all, the websites featured represent all different points of view.

National Food Safety Database
Website: http://www.foodsafety.org

Supported by the USDA and the Food Research Institute, this database has comprehensive information about a range of food safety topics, including links for storing and handling food; wild game; canning, drying, and freezing; people at high risk for foodborne illness; how foods can cause illness; microwave safety; product recalls; seafood safety; food safety for children; additives; and chemical residues. One of the most useful aspects of the site is the compilation of state experts and agencies.

North Carolina State University, Cooperative Extension Service, Food Safety Website
Website: www.ces.ncsu.edu/depts/foodsci/agentinfo

This website was designed by the cooperative extension service at NCSU to promote food safety by serving as a gateway site to other food safety sites. Information is divided into ten categories and the site has links to over 600 external sites as well as over 100 internal web pages. It can be searched by food type, cause of foodborne illness, or hot topics. Most of the page links are maintained by government agencies, extension services, and university food science departments and have detailed, practical information about food safety topics.

United States Food and Drug Administration, Center for Food Safety and Applied Nutrition, Foodborne Pathogenic Microorganisms and Natural Toxins Handbook (Bad Bug Book)
Website: http://vm.cfsan.fda.gov/~mow/intro.html

This is a comprehensive resource on the causes of foodborne illnesses. Each disease entry contains links to the Centers for Disease Control and Prevention's *Morbidity and Mortality Weekly Report*, which contains current outbreak information, and to the National Institutes of Health Medline database, which supplies current abstracts about the disease from medical journals. Each entry includes the nature of the disease, infective dose, associated foods, relative frequency of the disease, possible complications, target populations, and selected outbreaks. For a simplified version of the *Bad Bug Book*, go to http://www.agr.state.nc.us/cyber/kidswrld/foodsafe/badbug/badbug.htm.

Videotapes

All Hands on Deck! True Confessions of a Filthy, Rotten, Disgusting Germ
Date: 1996
Length: 10 minutes
Price: $25
Source: Brevis
            3310 South 2700 East
            Salt Lake City, UT 84109
            (800) 383-3377

A germ wearing a sweatshirt that says "SOAP KILLS" tells his family's secrets by explaining how and where germs linger in public restrooms. Thorough hand-washing technique is demonstrated, including how to avoid reinfection while turning off the water faucet and leaving the restroom. This funny video is appropriate for elementary school children and adolescents, as well as food service workers and consumers.

Are We Scaring Ourselves to Death?
Date: 1994
Length: 46 minutes
Price: $39.95
Source: ABC News
           P.O. Box 807
           New Hudson, MI 48165
           (800) 225-5222
           http://www.abcnews.com

In this interesting ABC News special, reporter John Stossel examines the fears of Americans, including crime, environmental pollution, food contamination, pesticides, and airplane crashes. He shows how manipulation of statistics and sensationalism by the media have made some risks look bigger than they really are. Stossel argues that by focusing on risks that are really quite small, we divert government attention and dollars from more substantial risks such as automobile accidents and how they could be better prevented. An intriguing table shows how much various risks shorten the average person's life.

Beagle Brigade
Date: 1994
Length: 12 minutes
Price: Free
Source: United States Department of Agriculture Office of
           Public Affairs
           4700 River Road
           Riverdale, MD 20737
           (301) 734-4895

This short, humorous documentary features the beagles of the U.S. Department of Agriculture that are used to aid the Animal and Plant Inspection Service at airports to detect food illegally brought into the United States. Beagles are used because they are friendly and their sense of smell is up to one thousand times more sensitive than that of humans. The entry of fruits and meats from other countries is heavily regulated to prevent insects from damaging U.S. crops or causing illness. This video can be viewed on the web at http://www.aphis.usda.gov/lpa/video/.

The Brain Eater

Date: 1998
Length: 60 minutes
Price: $19.95
Source: Public Broadcasting Company Home Video
P.O. Box 751089
Charlotte, NC 28275
(800) 949-8670

This *Nova* presentation explores bovine spongiform encephalopathy, otherwise known as mad cow disease, and its link to
Creutzfeldt-Jakob disease in humans. The disease is compared to
kuru, the neurological disease caused by cannibalism. Prions, the
deformed protein molecule that some think cause the disease, are
described. Scientists who agree with the prion theory and scientists who believe the disease is most likely viral are interviewed.

Case History Series

Date: 1985
Length: 10 minutes each, 9 tapes
Price: $245 for each video
Source: Altschul Group Corporation
1560 Sherman Avenue, Suite 100
Evanston, IL 60201
(800) 421-2363

Each tape reenacts a foodborne disease outbreak that originates in
a restaurant kitchen. The cause of the problem is clearly illustrated, the symptoms and consequences of the disease are
described, and ways of preventing the illness are presented. These
tapes are geared toward food service workers but would also be
useful to others interested in a visual demonstration of the contamination process. Titles include *Staphylococcus aureus (from sauces)*,
Staphylococcus aureus (from meats), *Hepatitis A*, *Bacillus cereus*,
Salmonella (from eggs), *Salmonella (from meat)*, *Campylobacter*, and
Clostridium botulinum.

Eating Defensively: Food Safety Advice for Persons with AIDS

Date: 1989
Length: 14.5 minutes
Price: $12
Source: U.S. Centers for Disease Control and Prevention
1600 Clifton Road, NE
Atlanta, GA 30333
(404) 639-3311

People with AIDS are up to three hundred times more likely to contract a foodborne illness, and foodborne illnesses are often fatal to immune-compromised individuals. This video guides the viewer through the kitchen, grocery store, restaurants, and even traveling abroad, explaining how to shop, store, cook, eat out, and travel safely. Although designed for AIDS patients, this video would be helpful for anyone who is immune compromised or who cooks for someone who is, such as chemotherapy patients and very elderly individuals.

The Eggs Games

Date: 1999
Length: 18 minutes
Price: $10
Source: American Egg Board
1460 Renaissance Drive
Park Ridge, IL 60068
(847) 296-7043

A slickly produced video, *The Eggs Games* simulates a sporting event complete with media coverage. Each individual competes in receiving, storing, and preparing eggs in a restaurant setting. The announcers describe the scoring process, which is based on proper egg-handling techniques. This video is an excellent example of how a trade organization can encourage the safe use of its product. Designed for food service workers.

Fast Track Food Safety Series
Date: 1994
Length: 5 tapes, each 20 to 25 minutes
Price: $499 for the set; may also be ordered individually
Source: Educational Institute of the American Hotel and
            Motel Association
            2113 N. High Street
            East Lansing, MI 48906
            (800) 344-4381

This series contains five tapes. The first, *Food Safety Essentials,* explains six food safety principles and subsequent videos focus on particular tasks in restaurants, including *Service, Warewashing, Food Production,* and *Receiving and Storing,* and how to properly implement the six principles when performing these tasks. The six principles are as follows: (1) Food safety starts with you. (2) Professionals prevent contamination. (3) Store smart. (4) Observe time and temperature guidelines. (5) Wash clean, rinse clear, and sanitize safely. (6) Watch out for warning signs. Foodborne illness is explained. A high-quality production with good graphics. Also available in Spanish.

Fight Bac! Keep Food Safe from Bacteria
Date: 1999
Length: 20 minutes
Price: Free to educators
Source: Partnership for Food Safety Education
            800 Connecticut Avenue NW, Suite 500
            Washington, DC 20006-2701
            (202) 429-8273

Designed as part of a curriculum unit for fourth through sixth graders, this video shows a foodborne illness outbreak that results from unsafe food handling at an after-school party. The video emphasizes safe food-handling techniques according to the rubric: Clean (clean hands and surfaces); Separate (keep foods separate; don't cross-contaminate); Cook (cook meats to proper temperatures); and Chill (refrigerate promptly). The storytelling vehicle is an effective way of conveying food safety facts.

Food Safe Series

Date: 1987
Length: 10 minutes each, 4 tapes in the series
Price: $245 each
Source: Altschul Group Corporation
1560 Sherman Avenue, Suite 100
Evanston, IL 60201
(800) 421-2363

This series covers general aspects of food safety with the goal of giving food safety workers both a theoretical and practical context for preventing foodborne illness. Each video covers a separate food safety topic. Titles include *Receiving and Storing, Facilities and Equipment, Microbiology for Food Service Workers,* and *Housekeeping and Pest Control.* The microbiology tape is appropriate for a more general audience and includes information about how beneficial bacteria is used in food production, for example, yogurt, as well as how harmful bacteria can get into the food supply.

Food Safety

Date: 1995
Length: 33 minutes
Price: $79
Source: Cambridge Educational
P.O. Box 2153
Charleston, WV 25328
(800) 468-4227

This video aimed at consumers demonstrates proper methods of buying, storing, preparing, and cooking food safely. The program hostess is lively, and interviews with an infectious disease specialist, a university extension agent, and a health department sanitarian reinforce key points. Examples from both a home and professional kitchen illustrate the universality of good food-handling practices. Commonsense techniques are stressed throughout the production.

Foodborne Illnesses and Their Prevention
Date: 1995
Length: 31 minutes
Price: $79
Source: Cambridge Educational
             P.O. Box 2153
             Charleston, WV 25328
             (800) 468-4227

This video geared toward the consumer or food service worker describes various foodborne illnesses, including symptoms, modes of transmission, and prevention. An interview with an epidemiologist and a microbiologist gives insight into bacteria, viruses, types of diseases, and how they spread. Procedures for preparing safe food are presented along with proper cooking temperatures. Very informative, if a little dry.

My Father's Garden
Date: 1995
Length: 58 minutes
Price: $250 purchase, $80 rental
Source: Bullfrog Films
             P.O. Box 149
             Oley, PA 19547
             (800) 543-3764

Two farmers are featured in this film, Fred Kirschenmann, an organic farmer in North Dakota, and Herbert Smith, an orange grower in Florida, who embraced the chemical fertilizers and pesticides that became available in the 1950s. Kirschenmann returned to his family farm in the 1970s and converted it to organic agriculture. To avoid using chemicals, Kirschenmann uses crop rotation and includes manure from cows he raises to improve the soil. Crop rotation benefits the soil by adding back nutrients and discouraging insects that like to feed on one crop all year. The film discusses the problems with chemical fertilizers, including health problems, topsoil erosion, and high prices. Interestingly, Kirschenmann has been able to make his farm economically viable with yields often better than when he was farming with chemicals.

Operation Safe Food
Date: 1994
Length: 3 tapes: 46 minutes, 71 minutes, 45 minutes
Price: $75
Source: University of Wyoming
CES P.O. Box 3354
Laramie, WY 82071
(307) 766-3379

Taped from a satellite video conference held in 1993, three experts including an extension agent, a food safety consultant specializing in implementing technical solutions to resolve food safety issues, and a health department inspector and trainer present each segment. This production is remarkable for the amount and depth of coverage it provides. The first speaker describes foodborne illnesses, gives case studies, and outlines HACCP. The second segment covers the changing trend from cook-serve to cook-chill where foods are cooked in advance, chilled, and served to patrons later. This process creates greater potential for foodborne illness than when foods are cooked and served immediately. The heat transfer process is thoroughly explained so the viewer can understand the reasons behind various cooling procedures. The third speaker covers personal habits, hygiene, and hand washing and how they affect food safety. A very informative and engaging presentation.

Pesticides and Pills: For Export Only, Part I, Pesticides
Date: 1981
Length: 57 minutes
Price: $99 or $149 for Parts I and II. (Part II is about expired and banned drugs exported overseas.)
Source: Robert Richter Productions
330 W. 42nd Street, 32nd Floor
New York, NY 10036
(212) 643-1208

Although this documentary was produced many years ago, pesticides banned in the United States are still being sold from the United States to Third World countries. As this documentary shows, at least half a million people worldwide are suffering from pesticide poisoning, a condition that results from direct exposure to pesticides in a field. This does not include increases in birth defects, miscarriages, genetic changes, or nutritional changes due to consumption of pesticides in foods. Less developed nations often lack the infrastructure to monitor and test pesticides in the way that the U.S. Environmental Protection Agency does. Pesticides are often sold without directions for use and with no caution labels. Ironically, many of these banned pesticides return to the United States and other developed nations in the form of pesticide residues. Fifty to 70 percent of pesticides used in less developed countries are on export crops. The U.S. Food and Drug Administration estimates that 10 percent of imported crops are contaminated with banned pesticides. However, there are many such pesticides that are undetectable with the methods used by the FDA, so the number is probably much higher.

Preventing Foodborne Illness

Date: 1996
Length: 10 minutes (includes 10 minutes each in English and Spanish)
Price: Free
Source: Colorado Department of Public Health and Environment
             Disease Control and Epidemiology Division
             4300 Cherry Creek Drive South
             Denver, CO 80222
             (303) 692-2700

Directed at food handlers, this video identifies three main causes of foodborne illness: failure to wash hands, failure to heat or cool foods adequately, and cross-contamination. Through demonstrations in a restaurant kitchen, proper hand washing, heating, cooling, and preparation techniques are shown to eliminate these hazards. Gloves are recommended for preparing foods that will not be cooked before serving or when the food handler has a cut. Workers are cautioned to stay home when sick. The tape comes with a useful summary that could be used as a reminder chart on a bulletin board.

Sanitizing for Safety
Date: 1990
Length: 17 minutes
Price: $12.95
Source: Clorox Company
1221 Broadway
Oakland, CA 94612
(888) 797-7225

Designed for food service workers, this video describes the main causes of foodborne illnesses, including improper personal hygiene, cross-contamination, and improper food handling and storage. The narrator notes that the average cost to a restaurant of an episode of foodborne illness is $74,000 in lost sales and medical and legal expenses. Preventative techniques are shown, including proper hand washing, storage techniques to minimize the time food is in the danger zone of 40 to 140 degrees, how to avoid cross-contamination, and how to sanitize cooking surfaces. Although there are other methods for sanitizing, this video demonstrates how to sanitize using bleach.

Save the Earth, Feed the World
Date: 1990
Length: 60 minutes
Price: $19.95
Source: Public Broadcasting Company Home Video
P.O. Box 751089
Charlotte, NC 28275
(800) 949-8670

Part of the Race to Save the Planet series, this video shows that not only has the "green revolution" of the 1960s failed to increase crop yields, but it has harmed the fertility of the soil, harmed people who work in the fields, and made consumption of crops more hazardous. Shot in the Central Valley of California, it describes a cancer cluster of farmworkers and their children, shows rice farming in Indonesia, and shows the effect of pesticides on wildlife, water, and children. On a hopeful note, methods that use fewer or no pesticides are beginning to make economic sense. In Indonesia, farmers are using integrated pest management, a method where pesticides are applied very selectively, along with other techniques like introducing beneficial insects, to control pests. An organic grain farmer in North Dakota has achieved comparable yields to those of conventional agriculture at a lower cost. A fresh produce company in Ventura, California, has made the switch to organic methods because it fills a market niche.

Serve Food Safely: A Volunteer Training System
Date: 1997
Length: 45 minutes
Price: $94.95
Source: Area Agency on Aging
1034 Park Avenue
Meadville, PA 16335
(800) 321-7705

This video and accompanying training manual is designed to help volunteers serve food safely in senior centers or other volunteer food service agencies such as churches, soup kitchens, and food delivery programs. According to the video, 20 percent of all emergency room visits are caused by foodborne illness. The videotape is divided into nine five-minute lessons that are reinforced with material in the manual: looking at the enemy, receiving, storage, preparation, cooking, serving, cooling and reheating, cleaning and sanitizing, and home-delivered meals. The video is shot in a volunteer food service setting and all the workers pictured are older adults.

Top Ten Causes of Foodborne Illness
Date: 1997
Length: 10 minutes
Price: $90 or $150 for the complete 50-minute series
Source: Drexel University
Food Safety First!
One Drexel Plaza, 3001 Market Street
Philadelphia, PA 19104

The maitre d' of Le Germ Café and Chef Ptomaine illustrate the top ten causes of foodborne illness and give the percentage of the time that they cause illness. They include improper cooling of cooked foods, overprepping (keeping food too long), not reheating food thoroughly, improper hot holding (not keeping food hot enough), dangerous food mixing, food from unsafe sources (homemade), improper cleaning of pots and utensils, and inadequate cleaning. The presentation is very entertaining. Although designed for food service workers, this material could apply to the home kitchen as well. This video is available by itself or with four other ten-minute segments, including personal hygiene and hand washing, cleaning and sanitation, preventing cross-contamination, and avoiding time and temperature abuse. Also available in Spanish.

Wash Your Hands
Date: 1995
Length: 5.5 minutes
Price: $65
Source: LWB Company
            13614 56th Avenue NE
            Marysville, WA 98271
            (360) 653-9122

In this short video geared toward consumers, food service workers, and adolescents, proper hand-washing technique is taught through the use of humor. Robert starts to leave the restroom when a mysterious voice reminds Robert to wash his hands. When Robert does a cursory job, the voice shows him microscopic evidence of the germs left on his hands and instructs him in proper hand-washing technique.

Glossary

active ingredient Substance in a product that performs the function of the product.

acute toxicity A toxic reaction that occurs shortly after exposure to a toxin (usually within a few hours or days).

adulterant Contaminant to a product added either intentionally to thin the product or unintentionally. Federal government prohibits adulterants in food.

aerobic Process that requires oxygen.

aerobic bacteria Bacteria that multiply in oxygenated environments.

anaerobic Absence of oxygen.

anaerobic bacteria Bacteria that multiply in an oxygen-free environment.

antibacterial cleanser A product designed to kill bacteria as well as clean.

assay Laboratory test or analysis.

bacteremia Blood disease caused when bacteria enters the bloodstream.

bacteria Single-celled organisms that multiply by dividing in two.

bioaccumulation The process by which a pesticide or other contaminant concentrates in higher amounts as it makes its way up the food chain.

bivalves Mollusks: clams, mussels, oysters. Animals with two shells hinged at one end.

BSE Bovine spongiform encephalopathy. A fatal neurological disease of cows. Also known as mad cow disease.

cancer Unregulated cell growth. Causes malignant tumors.

carbamates A class of synthetic pesticides that work by disrupting nerve function.

carcinogen A substance that causes cancer.

CDC Centers for Disease Control and Prevention. The U.S. government agency charged with investigating and preventing disease.

Codex Alimentarius International body that sets food standards to facilitate trade and promote food safety.

colonization Proliferation of bacteria in the gut.

competitive exclusion A system that introduces enough harmless bacteria into the gut of an animal to prevent bacteria that is harmful to humans from thriving.

contaminant Any substance, object, or germ that is in food and should not be.

cross-contamination Occurs when disease-causing organisms from one food (usually uncooked animal product) get onto another food. Usually occurs when foods are prepared on the same surface, or transferred by sponges, utensils, or aprons.

diarrhea Loose or watery bowel movements. Often caused by foodborne illness.

dose-response Occurs when there is a correlation between the amount of drug or toxin and its effect on health.

dysentery A diarrheal infection.

enteric infections Infections of the digestive system.

epidemiology The study of the incidence and distribution of disease or toxicity in human populations.

FAO Food and Agriculture Organization of the United Nations. The FAO works to improve agricultural practices, facilitate trade between nations, and improve the quality and quantity of the food supply.

FDA United States Food and Drug Administration. Responsible for regulating many foods and all drugs.

fecal-oral route Transfer of microorganisms from infected fecal matter on the hands to the digestive tract via the mouth. Usually occurs as a result of inadequate hand washing.

food poisoning An illness that occurs from eating a harmful food. This can be caused by chemicals, germs, or naturally occurring substances in the food.

foodborne illness An infectious disease caused by pathogens in food.

fungicide Chemicals used to kill or suppress fungi.

gamma radiation A type of radiation emitted from radioactive isotopes. Used to irradiate food.

gastroenteritis An inflammation of the stomach and intestinal tract that usually causes diarrhea.

genetically modified food Food developed by manipulating DNA.

HACCP (pronounced hassip) Hazard Analysis and Critical Control Points. A science-based system for improving food safety. Potential trouble spots are identified, and products are tested at various production points to ensure safety. This system is required for many food industries, and is widely used in most others.

herbicide Chemicals used to kill or suppress weeds.

HUS Hemolytic uremic syndrome. A serious complication of some foodborne illnesses including poisoning by *E. coli* O157:H7. The syndrome causes destruction of blood cells and then kidney damage when the shredded blood cells clog the kidneys.

illegal residue Presence of a pesticide or other substance at harvest in excess of the tolerance level.

immune compromised Person with a weakened immune system.

in vitro Literally, in glass. Studies or procedures carried out on cells or tissues in a test tube.

in vivo Literally, in life. Studies or procedures carried out on living animals or plants.

incubation period Length of time it takes to contract a disease after exposure.

infectious dose Number of bacteria, virus, or protozoa needed to cause disease.

insecticide Chemical used to kill insects.

IPM Integrated pest management. Use of two or more methods to control or prevent damage from pests. May include cultural practices (such as rotating crops), use of biological control agents (such as using beneficial insects to eat undesirable ones), and selective use of pesticides.

irradiation Treatment of food with low doses of radiation to kill or inactivate microorganisms.

kuru A fatal form of dementia caused by cannibalism. Specifically, a transmissible spongiform encephalopathy of the Fore people of New Guinea.

metabolite A compound derived by a chemical, biological, or physical action on a pesticide within a living organism. Metabolites can be more than, less than, or equally toxic as the original compound. Metabolites may also be produced by the action of environmental factors like sunlight and changing temperatures.

microbe Life-form only visible through a microscope. For example, bacteria, viruses, and protozoa.

microbial contamination In the case of food, food tainted with disease-carrying bacteria, parasites, or viruses.

microorganisms Life-forms only visible through a microscope. For example, bacteria, viruses, and protozoa.

mutagen A substance that causes changes (mutations) in the genetic traits passed from parent to offspring.

mycotoxins Toxins produced by fungi.

nematodes Wormlike organisms that inhabit the soil. They may also be a parasite on fish.

neurotoxins Chemicals that affect the nervous system. Severe reactions can include visual problems, muscle twitching, weakness, abnormalities of brain function, and behavioral changes.

offal Internal organs and soft tissue that are removed from a carcass when an animal is butchered.

oocyst Egg of a protozoa.

organochlorines Class of pesticides made by adding chlorine atoms to hydrocarbons. Includes DDT, dieldrin, and endrin. Used as insecticides. Persistent in the environment.

organophosphates Class of pesticides containing phosphorus. Kills insects by disrupting nerve function.

outbreak Two or more people contracting the same disease after exposure to the same microorganism.

parasite One organism that lives off another.

pasteurization Process for treating food by raising the temperature to a specific level and maintaining it for a set time to destroy microorganisms.

pathogen A microorganism that causes disease.

persistence The ability to remain in the environment for months or years without degrading into inert substances.

persistent pesticides Pesticides that remain in the environment for months or years without degrading into inert substances.

postmortem After-death examination of a body: autopsy.

protozoa Single-celled animals that live in soil or water.

radiolytic products Substances produced when food is irradiated.

rendered animal protein Leftovers from slaughtering plants and euthanized pets are sent to rendering plants where they are boiled (sometimes using vacuum technology at low temperatures) and dried.

residue Substance remaining in or on the surface of a food.

rodenticide   Chemical used to kill rodents such as mice, rats, and gophers.

ruminant-to-ruminant feeding   Process of feeding herbivores, like cows, animal products from a rendering plant.

serotype   A group of closely related microorganisms.

shelf life   Length of time a product is safe to eat as determined by the manufacturer and marked on the label.

shiga toxin   A poison released by certain types of bacteria including *E. coli* O157:H7.

stool   Bowel movement.

strain   A variant of a species member.

systemic pesticide   Pesticide that migrates to a different part of a plant or animal from which it was applied.

tolerance   Maximum amount of a substance legally allowed to contaminate a food.

toxins   Poisons produced by pathogenic bacteria.

verotoxins   Powerful toxins produced by some types of *E. coli.*

virulence   Degree to which bacteria can cause illness.

virus   A microbe is smaller than bacteria and needs a host cell to replicate.

Index

Nina E. Redman received her MLIS from San Jose State University. She is a librarian at Glendale College and Epson America. She is also the author of *Human Rights*, second edition, Contemporary World Issues (ABC-CLIO).